FALSE
POSITIVE

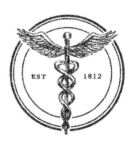

A Year of Error, Omission,
and Political Correctness in the

NEW ENGLAND
JOURNAL *of* MEDICINE

Theodore Dalrymple

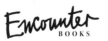
BOOKS

New York • London

First American edition published in 2019 by Encounter Books,
an activity of Encounter for Culture and Education, Inc.,
a nonprofit, tax exempt corporation.
Encounter Books website address: www.encounterbooks.com

Manufactured in the United States and printed on
acid-free paper. The paper used in this publication meets
the minimum requirements of ANSI/NISO Z39.48–1992
(R 1997) (*Permanence of Paper*).

FIRST AMERICAN EDITION

LIBRARY OF CONGRESS CATALOGING-IN-PUBLICATION DATA
Names: Dalrymple, Theodore, author.
Title: False positive : a year of error, omission, and political correctness
in the New England journal of medicine / by Theodore Dalrymple.
Description: New York : Encounter Books, 2019. |
Includes bibliographical references and index.
Identifiers: LCCN 2018060034 (print) | LCCN 2019000052 (ebook) |
ISBN 9781641770477 (ebook) | ISBN 9781641770460 (hardcover : alk. paper)
Subjects: | MESH: New England journal of medicine. |
Publication Bias | Periodicals as Topic
Classification: LCC R118.6 (ebook) | LCC R118.6 (print) |
NLM WZ 345 | DDC 610.72--dc23
LC record available at https://lccn.loc.gov/2018060034

To the Memory of Joseph Hartmann, M.D.
Cardiologist and kindred spirit

No head so headly can be given,
But error slippery will creep in.
For man without error scarcely be,
So that error exceedeth all diligency.

—Robert Recorde,
The Grounde of Artes, 1552

CONTENTS

Reading the *New England Journal of Medicine,*
January 12, 2017 – January 4, 2018

Introduction

Most doctors read medical journals for guidance in their practice and assume that the summary and conclusions at the end of articles are more or less justified by what goes before. After all, medical journals have editors whose job it is not only to select articles worthy of inclusion but also to eliminate obvious error. For most of my career, I believed that they did their job.

This is the belief, too, of most journalists who relay the results of medical research to the general public as if they were incontestable. Of necessity, perhaps, journalists take the summary and conclusions of scientific papers at face value, having neither the time nor the inclination to inquire much further. A straightforward or unequivocal scientific fact is journalistically more compelling than is a still-unanswered question. Likewise, a doubling of the risk of a disease is a more dramatic story than the extreme unlikelihood of contracting the disease in the first place, even at double the risk – a small detail that medical journals often omit.

Since my retirement from medical practice, I have had time to read journals with much closer attention and have come to realize just how flawed much of their content is. One cannot take accuracy or even veracity for granted, irrespective of how many eminent editors are on the masthead of a journal. The responsibility for detecting error is the reader's, and he must keep his mind open as much to what has been omitted as to what is included. Ever since Sir Arthur Conan Doyle, one of the most famous medical authors of all time, recorded the exploits and dicta of Sherlock Holmes, we have been aware that the silence of the dog that did not bark may be as eloquent as any barking could be. The more carefully I read medical papers, the more often the dog that did not bark in the nighttime seems to me an important lesson. What is not said is often very revealing, especially to suspicious minds like mine has become.

I was encouraged to write this book after my nephew Joseph, who is a medical student in Paris, asked my help before the examination that he was about to take in the proper, critical way to read a medical research paper. I was never taught this and wish that I had been. In trying to help him, I clarified my own ideas.[1]

The causes of error are multitudinous, and range from carelessness to dishonesty, from wishful thinking to outright corruption, with everything in between. Medical research relies on ever-more-complex statistics to conclude anything at all, and common sense is often the first victim of technical sophistication. But there is no such thing as a perfect paper that omits nothing, answers all possible questions and cannot be criticized on any ground.

In the following pages, I examine the contents of the *New England Journal of Medicine* over the course of a year. Along with the *Lancet*, it is the most important and influential general medical journal in the world. When it pronounces on social philosophy, as it often does, it reads like *Pravda*, not in the sense that it is Marxist-Leninist, of course, but in the sense that it takes its own attitudes so much for granted, as being so indisputably virtuous and true, that other viewpoints are rarely if ever expressed in its pages. The *Journal* is certainly not alone in this regard: the *Lancet* is, if anything, worse. The dead hand of political correctness is upon medical journals.

My object has been twofold: first, to alert readers to the sickly self-righteousness that seems to me to have infected the *New England Journal of Medicine*, contracted no doubt from the wider culture; and second, to attune them to the ambiguities of the medical research that is so often taken to provide unequivocal answers, even to questions that are inescapably ethical in nature. It is not my wish to hold up anyone to ridicule or contempt, which is why I have omitted the names of

---

1 He passed the exam, but I do not want to fall into the old fallacy that because *a* followed *b* in time, *b* caused *a*.

authors, and only occasionally have inferred or ascribed motives when they seemed obvious to me.

I begin with the issue of January 12, 2017, because my annual subscription started on this date, and proceed week by week through January 4, 2018. My hope is that readers will come to see how complex and difficult medical research is, and how they should remain skeptical of medical findings reported in the general media. ◾

January 12, 2017

Not everyone, I suspect, would turn beating heart to an article with the title "Eliminating Cholera Transmission in Haiti," the first in the *Journal* this week. Haiti is of small account in the world, an infamously hopeless case of political pathology; but as I have twice visited the country, nothing Haitian is alien to me. The country grips the imagination of the visitor as no other; your passion for it, though it may fade a little with time, is rekindled at the first mention of its name. Its tragic destiny is like a highly compressed history of humanity, or a *memento mori* for the whole of mankind.

Nevertheless, there was good news in the article: two effective oral vaccines against cholera have been produced, one in India and one in South Korea (a sign of the shift of the world's scientific center of gravity, perhaps). I remember the days when cholera vaccines had to be injected in the upper arm and caused considerable soreness, though not necessarily much immunity to cholera. The new oral vaccines are stable for a month at 37 degrees Celsius, and therefore require no chain of refrigeration to be used successfully in remote rural areas. In Haiti, electricity is less reliable than the weather.

The second paragraph of an otherwise excellent article was almost as interesting for what it did *not* say as for what it did. Its first sentence informs us: "Cholera had not been recorded in Haiti until it was introduced in 2010." We then learn that the epidemic involved 800,000 cases, which is about 8 percent of the population, and that it resulted in 10,000 deaths. (A death rate of one in eighty cases demonstrates that even in

Haiti modern medical care has a long reach and a beneficial effect, for the death rate of cholera when it first appeared in Western countries in the nineteenth century was about 50 percent. We lament the state of the world, but progress, however uneven, has been patent.)[1]

But notice the dog that did not bark: cholera *was introduced*. By what, or by whom, was it introduced? Surely this is a matter of some interest and worth a word or two. Is the omission a sign of embarrassment?

The scientific evidence strongly suggests that cholera was introduced into Haiti by Nepali troops of the United Nations peacekeeping mission there, known by its initials MINUSTAH (Mission des Nations Unies pour la stabilisation en Haiti). Just before a group of them arrived in the country in October 2010, there had been an outbreak of cholera in Nepal, but no one thought to take precautionary measures to prevent the troops spreading the disease to Haiti, a place very vulnerable to any epidemic disease favored by poverty and poor or nonexistent sanitation. It seems that the sanitary arrangements for peacekeeping troops were so poor that soon after their arrival at a camp near the Artibonite River (Haiti's largest), a truck disposed of the soldiers' waste straight into the river. It provoked an epidemic that has not yet ended.

Needless to say, no one intended to start an epidemic of cholera in Haiti; but once it had started, a considerable effort went into covering up its source. The American Centers for Disease Control, the World Health Organization, the United Nations and various supposedly independent researchers went in for obfuscation until the evidence became almost undeniable that the Nepali peacekeeping troops had brought it with them.[2] Interestingly, the obfuscators were assisted in their obfuscation by the two most influential general medical journals in the world, the

---

1 It is necessary to be a little cautious in tracing the death rates from cholera because of different definitions of cases. Most people who are infected with the causative organism, *Vibrio cholerae*, do not suffer from the disease. They are cases of cholera infection, but not of cholera. The death rate therefore depends very considerably on case definition.

2 Nepali troops have been prominent in United Nations peacekeeping missions since 1959. The tradition continued even during the civil war in Nepal that lasted from 1996 to 2008. Thanks to Nepal's poverty, the troops are cheap and there has always been a large discrepancy between what the troops receive in pay and what the Nepali army receives from the United Nations. For Nepal, therefore, peacekeeping is a valuable source of income.

Lancet and the *New England Journal of Medicine*, both of which refused to publish scientific papers that made a very strong case that the Nepali soldiers were the source of the epidemic. The *Lancet* did, however, publish an article to the effect that speculating on the source of the epidemic was unnecessary and even counterproductive.

Why all the obfuscation? One can only guess. For one thing, the Haitian population, victim already of so many disasters both natural and political, was understandably angry when it first came to suspect that the Nepali troops were the source of the epidemic. There were some anti-Nepali riots, and the authorities feared that an admission of MINUSTAH's responsibility might lead to an explosion. Then, the longer they obscured the truth, the more difficult it was to admit. Who, in any case, likes to own up to having caused a catastrophe, even inadvertently? There was probably also a reluctance to believe that those who intended good could actually do harm, and on such a major scale. No one likes to think that the best of intentions can result in disaster, and so truth was avoided and untruth propagated.[3]

The *NEJM* certainly did not cover itself in glory during the whole episode, perhaps because it toed official lines. I surmise that the failure to mention who introduced cholera into Haiti (which after all would have taken no more than four words) was a sign of unease or even bad conscience among the editors, who normally lose no opportunity to put the *Journal's* humanitarian heart upon its sleeve.

Telling the truth would threaten not just a few individuals and institutions, but an entire worldview that was more difficult and painful to give up than a bad habit. No one could be against the United Nations; it would be like favoring cruelty over kindness. Alas, this was not the first time that an agency of the United Nations caused a catastrophe and then tried to cover it up.

In the 1970s, UNICEF and the World Bank attempted to reduce the very high infant mortality rate in Bangladesh by drilling millions of tube wells to provide bacteriologically clean groundwater. (A high percentage of infant deaths were caused by fecally contaminated

---

3 For a brilliant and riveting account of the affair, see Ralph R. Frerichs, *Deadly River: Cholera and Cover-Up in Post-Earthquake Haiti* (Ithaca, N.Y.: Cornell University Press, 2016).

surface water containing the agents of fatal gastroenteritis.) As far as reducing the infant mortality rate is concerned, the wells were a great success, but unfortunately the groundwater contained a high concentration of arsenic, a carcinogen. The result was that tens of millions of Bangladeshis now face the prospect of various kinds of cancer, from which thousands have already died. When this became evident, UNICEF tried for a long time to conceal it—a normal human reaction, no doubt, but not one to be expected of a humanitarian organization with no thought of self-interest.

〜

A review article titled "Screening for Colorectal Cancer" was of some personal interest to me because mine is a family in which this disease is frequent. In essence I read it to find some reason, or rather a rationalization, *not* to undergo the regular screening colonoscopy whose discomfort I fear. My eyes alighted at once upon a passage that fed my wishes:

> Although not all trials have shown a significant benefit with respect to reducing mortality...several large, randomized controlled trials have confirmed the effectiveness of one-time and periodic...sigmoidoscopy, with a 26 to 31% lower mortality from colorectal cancer....

So a regular colonoscopy appears to lower the death rate from colorectal cancer, but the paper never mentions the *all-cause* death rate. Thus it leaves open the possibility that screening might save people from dying of colorectal cancer, only for them to die of something else at the same age. What I want to know is whether screening is likely to extend my life, not just prevent me from dying of colorectal cancer. This is an important consideration if a disease is not especially common by comparison with other possibly fatal conditions.

I would also want to know the *absolute* risk of dying from colorectal cancer, not merely the reduction in *relative* risk. This is because a large reduction in relative risk may translate into a trivial reduction in absolute risk if the condition is rare to begin with, while a smaller reduction in the relative risk of a common condition may be much greater in absolute terms.[4] I am not saying that this is the case here, but the paper gives no means of working out the absolute risk. I have long made it a principle to mistrust papers where only relative and not absolute risks are given, or that make it very difficult to calculate the reduction in the absolute risk.

By its omissions, the paper gave me just what I wanted, then: a reason not to be screened.

⌒

Since writing this, I have had the opportunity (March 2019) to read Professor Renaud Piarroux's book, *Choléra: Haiti 2010–2018 histoire d'un désastre* (CNRS Éditions). From this it appears that, having followed the *NEJM*, I have considerably underestimated the cholera epidemic's lethality, perhaps as much as by eight times. ▣

---

4 Suppose that I have a one in a million chance of dying of disease X, and that by eating broccoli every day I can reduce the risk to one in three million. That is a reduction by two-thirds, but not very significant in absolute terms. It would hardly be worth the effort.

January 19, 2017

"Behind mountains, more mountains," say the peasants of Haiti. The more things are transparent, the more they are opaque; or perhaps they simply raise further difficult questions.

An article titled "Transparency and Trust—Online Patient Reviews of Physicians" raised more questions than it answered. The author, in impeccably bureaucratic prose, extols the potential value of reviews of doctors by patients, published on the internet:

> Patient reviews offer clinicians valuable performance feedback for learning and improving, both individually and across a system. Receptivity to performance feedback, which depends heavily on physicians' acceptance of the data's validity, facilitates a culture of continuous learning and patient-centeredness.

Note that what is yet to be proved is here taken to be established fact: what is surmised to be possibly or desirably the case actually *is* the case. I have sat through many meetings, and read many documents, in which bureaucrats have made precisely this assumption. The world, I have found, is often refractory to the best of intentions (the worst being easier to fulfill).

"Whenever I hear the word culture," Goering is reputed to have said, "I reach for my Browning [pistol]." Whenever I read bureaucratic prose, if any meaning at all can be discerned in it, I reach for my objections. Sometimes a still small voice whispers somewhere in the back of my head (it really feels located there) that my objections to whatever is proposed are really a manifestation of fear and dislike of change. The particular change discussed in this article hardly matters to me now that I am retired, but I wouldn't have wanted to know what my patients thought of me.

What are my objections to such internet reviews, which treat doctors as if they were restaurants? Among them are the possibility that patients may value the wrong things in their doctors. A patient is not a customer, and a doctor is not merely a provider of a service, like a shopkeeper who sells whatever his customers wish to purchase from his stock; he is very importantly an adviser also. A doctor may decline to do what his patient wants of him because he considers it not in the patient's interests. This might not win him a good review from the patient; but on the other hand, Dr. Harold Shipman was generally well regarded by his patients, and he turned out to be the most prolific serial killer in British history.

My wariness of online reviews was not entirely allayed by the three examples evaluating a surgeon named Courtney L. Scaife that were cited in the article. These reviews read:

1. Was thoroughly impressed with the physician.
2. Dr. Courtney is an excellent surgeon, she explains things very clearly, is very detailed and just amazing. I would recommend Dr. Scaife very highly.
3. It did feel like the provider is not as concerned for my condition as I am.

There is very little of any substance in these comments. One can easily be impressed by charlatans; indeed, whole books, often very amusing, have been written about the gullibility of humans, sometimes many thousands of people at once. Then too, only the survivors of surgery can give a review of their surgeon, so a doctor could decimate a countryside and receive glowing reports.

As for the critical remark among the three, would you trust the judgment of someone who wanted or expected his doctor to be "as concerned for my condition as I am"? A doctor who was concerned for his patient in precisely the same way and to the same degree as the patient was concerned for himself would be useless or worse, possibly dangerous. The doctor should be sympathetic, of course, and empathetic as well; but his sympathy and empathy for his patient are not those of the close friend or relative. The doctor is concerned for his patient but also detached from him, otherwise he would soon find himself paralyzed by emotion. A doctor cannot and should not grieve over the death of his patient in the way that a spouse, a child or a parent grieves. Not all is callous that is unemotional.

The comment that Dr. Scaife was not as concerned with her patient's condition as was the patient himself is an example of our increasing reluctance to draw proper distinctions, such as that between the appropriate and inappropriate use of the demotic, or of the formal and the informal. Gone is the understanding taught in Ecclesiastes: "To everything there is a season.... A time to weep, and a time to laugh.... A time for silence, and a time to speak...."

It is quite possible that Dr. Scaife was right in viewing the patient's condition as medically trivial and nothing worth worrying about, but this thought simply did not enter the patient's head.[1]

∽

Further on in the *Journal* is a paper titled "'Zombie' Outbreak Caused by the Synthetic Cannabinoid AMB-FUBINACA in New York," which tells us:

> On July 12, 2016, a synthetic cannabinoid caused mass intoxica-tions of 33 persons in one New York City neighborhood, in an event described in the press as a "zombie" outbreak because of the appear-ance of the intoxicated persons.

This is part of the latest chapter in man's eternal struggle to tune in, turn on and drop out. Hundreds of synthetic cannabinoids, the active ingredients of cannabis, are now being manufactured in clandestine laboratories around the world, but principally in China. In 2014 alone, 177 new cannabinoids were found to have been used in America. Not

---

1 I bear in mind, however, the dictum of Sir George Pickering, an eminent British physician, that a minor operation is an operation performed on somebody else.

surprisingly, the authorities have difficulty in keeping up with the ingenuity and dedication of the chemists.

The attraction of the synthetic cannabinoids, for those who manufacture and distribute them, is that they are highly potent, easy to
smuggle and saleable in tiny quantities at enormous profit. The
attraction for those who take them is less obvious, since the effects
are distinctly unpleasant and sometimes dangerous, ranging from
lightheadedness to psychosis, delirium, fits, kidney failure and death
(though the danger may actually increase the attraction for a certain
kind of person). A variant of the drug that was the subject of this paper,
AMB-FUBINACA, was recognized in a product called Trainwreck #2,
sold in Louisiana, and is described on websites devoted to discussions
of drugs as *out of this world potent*. Both the name and the description
are indications of the mental nihilism of those who would take the
drug. The product that caused the zombification of the thirty-three
people in New York was called AK-47 24 Karat Gold. What's in a
name? Sometimes quite a lot.

It might be supposed that some more obviously pleasurable effects
would induce people to take drugs. In some cases this is no doubt so,
but by no means always. In the prison in which I worked as a doctor,
prisoners who found a cache of pills would take them all, without
the faintest knowledge of what they were or what effects they would
have. The hope was for oblivion, or at least a change in mental state,
though not necessarily an improvement. (Sometimes they ended up
being hospitalized.) This proclivity is not unique to prison inmates,
of course. I have often heard young British people discuss their wonderful previous night, the proof of how good it was being that, thanks
to the alcohol they consumed, they could remember nothing about it.
Oblivion was the highest pleasure available to them. In the Gilbert
Islands, in the Central Pacific, I asked young people why they deliberately sniffed the fumes of petrol, whose effects were nausea, dizziness,
severe headache, impaired coordination and, eventually, unconscious-
ness—not pleasant effects on the face of it. They replied that petrol
fumes made them feel *different*. Their lives, it was true, were monoto-
nous, there being no seasons and the day lasting twelve hours all year
round; they desired difference in their state of mind even at the cost
of considerable discomfort. And on the island of Ibiza, where at least

some of the youth of Europe like to spend their holidays, the two enormous nightclubs, with room for thousands, are called Manumission and Amnesia, as if only forgetfulness could bring release from slavery.

The "zombie" outbreak in New York thus fell into a sad saga of efforts to escape the mundane. The good news is that the identification and chemical characterization of the drug that caused the zombification—the blank stare and lead-pipe movements of an early Hollywood science-fiction humanoid—took only seventeen days and was a technical and organizational triumph, as the *Journal* reports:

> Collaboration among clinical laboratory staff, health professionals, and law enforcement agencies facilitated the timely identification of the compound and allowed health authorities to take appropriate action.... This type of coordination among multiple agencies is important for the timely resolution of future outbreaks.

Unfortunately, however, the paper gives no indication of what such *resolution* consists of, or what the health authorities' appropriate action might be. An outlawing of human stupidity, perhaps?

↶

A review article with the title "Mechanisms, Pathophysiology, and Management of Obesity" informs us that "People who are overweight or obese account for more than two thirds of the U.S. population and are overrepresented in primary care practices." This would mean that the great majority of American patients in primary care, presumably three-quarters at least, are fat.

The explanation offered for this lamentable fact of modern America is interesting for what it does not say:

> Factors favoring a positive energy balance and weight gain over the past several decades include increasing per capita food supplies and consumption, particularly of high-calorie, palatable foods that are often served in large portions;...and displacement of leisure-time activities with sedentary activities such as television watching and use of electronic devices.

The culprits, then, would be our old friends, two of the Deadly Sins: greed and sloth. But it cannot be put so forthrightly. "Speak not in the ears of a fool: for he will despise the wisdom of thy words." ▣

January 26, 2017

I fondly imagined that I was up to date with the acronyms pertaining to sex and gender, until I saw an article titled "Intimate Choices, Public Threats—Reproductive and LGBTQ Rights under a Trump Administration." What did the *Q* stand for? Eventually I learned that it stood for *queer*. But surely *queer* was already covered by the G for *gay*? No further explanation was forthcoming.

I realized that I was already behind the times, even though I had read an article in the *Journal* just a few months earlier explaining the new, *correct* sexual terminology. Nowadays we have cis- and trans-gender, as in the old days we had Cis- and Trans-Jordan. The article listed something called *genderqueer*, a term apparently in such common use already that my Word program, thanks to repeated updates, does not underline it with a red wavy line, as it does when it thinks I have made a spelling mistake. A genderqueer person is one who identifies as both male and female, or neither. But Q can hardly stand for the *genderqueer*, unless that term has been shortened to *queer* in the interval. The article on terminology cautioned that its own list was not definitive, for as it delicately put it, "concepts are evolving." They certainly are.

In any case, the acronym LGBTQ struck me as outrageously noninclusive. Surely it should, at the very least, be LGBTQFNPI, standing for Lesbian, Gay, Bisexual, Transsexual, Queer, Fetishist, Necrophiliac, Polygamist, Incestophile? Even this, as readers of Krafft-Ebing's *Psychopathia Sexualis* will appreciate, by no means exhausts the possibilities: an acronym truly reflective of human sexual variety would be several pages long.

Be that as it may, the more recent article is not about taxonomy but about "rights." Most articles in the medical press that discuss rights seem to me to confuse two uses of the word *right*, and this statement in the *Journal* is typical: "The Hyde Amendment limits the use of Medicaid funds for abortion procedures, preventing poor women from exercising their constitutional rights." Leaving aside the question whether the United States Constitution either permits or forbids abortion (I suspect that it does neither), note that the statement assumes that the exercise of a right requires not just an absence of restraint but also, in some cases, the provision of benefits.

But saying that I have a right (correctly understood) to eat chocolate does not in the least mean that anyone has a duty to supply me with chocolate or to ensure that chocolate is available to me. My right to eat chocolate is not infringed by an absence of chocolate to eat. Likewise, failing to make public funds available for abortion procedures does not abrogate anyone's right to an abortion.

A regime of proliferating "rights," defined to include claims on the provision of goods, has the tendency to stultify the moral imagination. Where something is granted as of right, there is no necessity to think of any other reason why it should be granted. When I ask students why people should be given health care, they generally cannot think of any reason other than "people have a right to it." For them, it is a right, or it is nothing.

❧

There has been a marked tendency of late for the *Journal* to publish negative results, that is to say, results of experiments in which the treatment being tested has not worked. This trend toward more negativity is actually a positive development, a corrective to the *publication bias* following from a longstanding preference for positive results.

The January 26 issue published negative results involving the use of hypothermia (reduced body temperature) in the treatment of cardiac arrest in children while they are in hospital. A cardiac arrest stops blood flow to the brain, and when it is restored, there is quite often permanent brain damage. In adults it has been found that cooling the body after cardiac arrest reduces the brain damage, presumably because lowering the metabolic demand reduces the difference between what is needed and what is available. If it works in adults, the reasoning went, why should it not work in children?

There is, however, no more dangerous argument in medicine than *It stands to reason*, since what stands to reason may not be so in fact. For hundreds of years, if not thousands, what stood to reason on the basis of the humoral theory of disease was assiduously practiced, almost certainly doing more harm than good. It may stand to reason that what works in one group of people should work in another, but this is often not the case, which is one of the reasons why it is necessary to avoid drawing conclusions too widely from a single experiment. Indeed, the results of transferring conclusions from one group of patients to another may be disastrous (as we will see later concerning the prescription of opiates for pain).

The experiment using hypothermia in children was conducted in thirty-seven hospitals; it had to be conducted in so many hospitals because cardiac arrest in children is not very common. Here is a summary of what was done and the results:

> Within 6 hours after the return of circulation, comatose children older than 48 hours and younger than 18 years of age were randomly assigned to therapeutic hypothermia (target temperature 33.0°C) or therapeutic normothermia (target temperature, 36.8°C)....The trial was terminated because of futility after 329 patients had undergone randomization....Among children who survived in-hospital cardiac arrest, therapeutic hypothermia, as compared with therapeutic normothermia, did not confer a significant benefit in survival with a favorable functional outcome at 1 year.

A vast effort for nothing, it might seem. (The paper names no fewer than forty-nine authors!) But appearances can be deceptive. It is as necessary to know that a procedure does not work, or causes harm, as that it does work—all the more so when it is expensive and time-consuming.

The failure to publish negative results, especially in the field of pharmacology, can give a misleading impression of a medication's efficacy. If, for example, there were ten trials of a new medication, only one of which found it to be effective, failing to publish the results of the other nine trials would lead doctors to suppose that it *was* effective, though if all the results were amalgamated, it would be shown not to be effective. Before this was understood, medical journals skewed toward positive results, and this bias has real consequences for practice.

This is one of the reasons why in many countries it is now legally obligatory for all medical trials to be registered with a central registry, for their protocols to be published in advance and for their results to be published, if only online. Moreover, trials are supposed to be registered as soon as they start, if not beforehand, so that those who conduct them do not change their aims as they go along if it becomes clear that their original aims will not be met. This is important, because if you generate a lot of data you can always derive some kind of result from them; but to do so is not scientifically legitimate. Suppose you correlate the consumption of two hundred different foods with car crashes: you are bound to find a positive or negative correlation or two, perhaps a correlation with the consumption of apples. But this is a nearly worthless finding, unless backed up by further experiment to establish that the correlation was reproducible. Only if the collection of data is preceded by a hypothesis is any conclusion from it likely (though not certain) to be valid.

Another article in the *Journal* this week describes the work of the American registry of trials that has been in operation since 2000. I was astonished to see that 208,822 such trials have been registered during that time (and 323,018 in the World Health Organization's registry, 208,024 of them overlapping with the American registry). This shows how vast is now the enterprise of medical research. The article does not tell us how much of this enterprise, including the registry itself, contributes to progress. The question, though a real one, is unanswerable.

It has long been thought that good, honest research is impeded by the commercial interest that funds it. In the medical field, this essentially means the drug companies. Of course, researchers have interests to promote other than commercial ones. They may be so attached to a favorite theory that they bend results in the interest of what they perceive to be the higher truth; or they may desire good results for purely careerist reasons. Authors are now asked to declare their possible pecuniary interests and paid work for drug companies, on the assumption that if they do so they will not bend their results at the behest of their paymasters. In a trial of a new drug published in this week's *Journal*, financed by a drug company, one of the authors declared that he has received:

consulting fees from Alere, Actelion Pharmaceuticals, Cubist Pharmaceuticals, Astellas, Optimer Pharmaceuticals, Sanofi Pasteur, Summit Pharmaceuticals, bioMérieux, Da Volterra, Qiagen, Cerexa, Abbott, AstraZeneca, Pfizer, Durata Therapeutics, Merck, Seres Therapeutics, Valneva, Nabriva Therapeutics, Roche, the Medicines Company, and Basilea Pharmaceutica, lecture fees from Actelion Pharmaceuticals, Cubist Pharmaceuticals, Astellas, Optimer Pharmaceuticals, Sanofic Pasteur, Summit Pharmaceuticals, bioMérieux, Da Volterra, Qiagen, AstraZeneca, and Pfizer, and grant support from Alere, Actelion Pharmaceuticals, Cubist Pharmaceuticals, Astellas, Optimer Pharmaceuticals, Sanofi Pasteur, Summit Pharmaceuticals, bioMérieux, Da Volterra, Qiagen, Cerexa, and Abbott.

It might have saved space to list those companies that had *not* paid him consulting fees, for whom he had *never* lectured, and that had *not* financed his research.

And before one says, oh well, that's America for you, I note that the author was English, working in England. ◾

February 2, 2017

In Samuel Butler's satire, *Erewhon* (an anagram of Nowhere, that is to say, nowhere *yet*), criminals are treated as ill and the ill as criminals. The question of moral responsibility is always a contested one, and no one is such a determinist that he never blames anyone for anything. Indeed, the human desire to blame people is at least as strong as the desire to excuse them and to regard them as the helpless victims of circumstance. In view of the complexity of human existence, people are not simply guilty or innocent, but often something in between the two (which is why decent legal systems recognize mitigating circumstances).

There is a reminder of moral complexity in an article that is part of a series called "Clinical Problem Solving." The patient whose problem was to be solved was "a 49-year-old man with a weight of 159 kilos (350 pounds) and a body-mass index...of 49.1" who presented for bariatric (weight-reducing) surgery. This man, we are informed, "had been morbidly obese since childhood." In other words, he had been fed far too much early in life, and probably the wrong things, certainly before the age of discretion. Everyone in the field is agreed that it is easier to remain slim than to become slim after having been fat. This is not to say that it is impossible to do the latter, by eating less. But it would be a very censorious person who made no allowances for this man as far as responsibility for his plight is concerned.

Another article this week deals more broadly with medical conditions that arise from the patient's actions. Titled "Medicare Payment for Behavioral Health Integration," it begins:

> Integrating behavioral health care with primary care is now widely
> considered an effective strategy for improving outcomes for the many
> millions of Americans with mental or behavioral health conditions.

Let us overlook the question of who is doing the considering here.
What are the *behavioral health conditions* from which so many millions
of Americans suffer? They include the old favorites: drinking too much,
smoking, taking drugs, and obesity, which is a consequence of eating
too much, undoubtedly a behavior.

The medical consequences of obesity are legion, and include Type 2
diabetes, the prevalence of which is of epidemic proportions, and which
some epidemiologists believe will reverse the continuous increase in
life expectancy of the last century and a half. Another consequence is
accelerated osteoarthritis: it is not uncommon to see very fat people
in wheelchairs, crippled at an early age by arthritis resulting from the
weight that their joints have to bear. Because eating too much is the
cause of obesity, and eating too much is behavioral, it seems *prima facie*
plausible to call conditions such as Type 2 diabetes and osteoarthritis
behavioral—all the more so since the former, at least, tends to remit if
the patient loses weight by whatever means.

These conditions are to be treated by means of *behavioral health
integration*. That term has a distinctly dystopian ring, conjuring up
mental images of electric shocks to extinguish bad habits and replace
them by docility, à la *Clockwork Orange*. Other behavioral treatments
in the past included giving apomorphine to opiate addicts to make
them vomit when they took opiates, in the hope that it would set
up a conditioned response such that they would feel nausea at the
very sight of opiates without having to be given the apomorphine to
induce it. This article proposes nothing so drastic, but it suggests
that behavioral health integration is economically efficient as well as
clinically effective:

> Widespread implementation of CoCM [the Psychiatric Collaborative
> Care Model] and other effective BHI [Behavioral Health Integration]
> could substantially improve outcomes for millions of Medicare ben-
> eficiaries and produce savings for the Medicare program.

The evidence for this assertion (which the authors, to their credit, at least keep to the conditional mood) is that various trials have shown those acronymic procedures to be effective. Entirely overlooked is the well-known fact that the results of trials, which are usually conducted with care and with the enthusiasm of participants, do not necessarily translate into what is known as the real world, in day-to-day practice, especially in a field where the outcomes are relatively ill defined and therefore easy to fake.

To me, it all sounds typical of bureaucratic appeals to spend money in order to save it in the end (rather like saving villages by destroying them). The expenditures are always certain, the economies always hypothetical. Before long, boredom supervenes and one's eyes begin to glaze over:

> Using...three new codes, the primary care physician can bill Medicare for each month in which a threshold amount of time is spent delivering CoCM services (for the first month, approximately $140 for 70 minutes per beneficiary; for subsequent months, approximately $125 for 60 minutes per beneficiary; and for all months, approximately $65 for each additional 30 minutes per beneficiary). The behavioral health care manager must have formal education or specialized training in behavioral health....

To make absolutely sure that the reader's mind is numbed into submission, the article continues in this vein:

> Since CoCM is not the only approach to BHI in use today, Medicare will also begin making separate payments using a fourth new code for services furnished according to other BHI models (approximately $48 for at least 20 minutes of services per beneficiary per month). This code can be used to report services provided under other BHI care models that include systematic assessment and monitoring using validated clinical rating scales (where applicable), behavioral health care planning (with care plan revision for patient whose condition is not improving), facilitation and coordination of behavioral health treatment....

In practice this will boil down to a lot of form filling, a completed form being regarded by the *behavioral health worker* as an achievement in itself. As for *facilitation and coordination,* they are usually work-creation schemes for facilitators and coordinators.

Toward the end of his life, Sigmund Freud wrote a paper titled "Analysis, Terminable and Interminable." I was reminded of it in observing that nothing in the description of CoCM and BHI suggests any limits to payments for them. Without such limits, they are likely to be interminable. Ineffectiveness will be rewarded: and in this field there is plenty of ineffectiveness to reward. ▣

February 9, 2017

Two articles tackle the important but vexed question of how best to pay doctors for their services, especially those who take care of the least well-off patients. The articles start with such strikingly similar paragraphs that for a moment I thought I was reading the first article for a second time. The first begins:

> Medicare is steadily shifting from volume-based fee-for-service to value-based payment models....

And the second:

> The United States is rapidly moving to a health care delivery system in which value-based payment models are the predominant way of reimbursing clinicians for care.

The two statements are subtly different, however. Is the shift *steady* but the movement *rapid?* I suppose that strictly speaking there is no contradiction between them—you can locomote at a steady but rapid pace—though normally the words have a different connotation. As a person approaching old age, I think I would prefer a steady decline to a rapid one, if decline there must be.

The first of the articles is titled "Social Risk Factors and Equity in Medicare Payment." The word *equity* is here (for once) used correctly, to mean fairness, not equality. Under consideration is the comparative fairness of a fee-for-service versus a results-based payment system.

Fee-for-service is equitable in the sense that the more doctors do, the more they are paid. The characteristics of the recipients of their services do not affect what they are paid; a blood test is a blood test, after all. But there is a problem with fee-for-service remuneration: it takes no account of whether or not the service paid for was necessary, whether or not it benefited the patient. Unnecessary tests and operations are done in large numbers and add considerably to the cost of health care while swelling the income of doctors. This is not necessarily dishonesty on the doctor's part, at least not of a crude kind, even if it sometimes is. It is easy for a doctor to persuade himself that a test is necessary just as a precaution, and a monetary incentive will tip the balance in its favor if he is ambivalent about the need to do it.

Payment-by-results eliminates or reduces the incentive to perform unnecessary tests or procedures, especially if value-for-money is part of the calculation. But payment-by-results is not as easy, or as fair, as it sounds. For payment-by-results to be fair, like must be compared with like. For example, it is well known that the results of operations performed on fat smokers are less good than those of operations on slim nonsmokers (being fat is the new norm in the United States), and good results are harder to achieve among the lower socioeconomic strata than among the higher. Therefore, to pay doctors according to their results irrespective of the characteristics of their patients would be unfair, and furthermore it would have the effect (already noticeable enough) of encouraging doctors to congregate in rich areas or practices and spurn the poor.

Ensuring equity of payment in the article's meaning (fairness to the doctors who do the work) thus requires the gathering of a great deal of data. And do you measure the characteristics of the population from which the doctor draws his patients, or only those of the patients he actually sees, which may not be at all the same, on average? The article doesn't say. In any case, while the gathering of data is often treated as if it were cost-free, it is not, as every modern doctor who spends much of his time inputting data of various kinds well knows. Sometimes it seems as if you can either know what you're doing, but not do very much, or do a lot without knowing what you are doing.

Which of the alternatives is better depends on the skill and probity of the doctor.

The second of the articles on the subject of payment to doctors takes the characteristics of patients into consideration, but applies a different understanding of *equity*. It is titled "Should Value-Based Purchasing Take Social Risk into Account?" The authors say that improved data collection and statistical techniques are needed to "measure and report quality of care for beneficiaries with social risk factors," and they continue:

> Another important component of this strategy is to measure equity itself. Health equity measures or domains should be developed and introduced into existing payment programs to measure disparities and provide incentives for reducing them.

Here, *health equity* seems to mean inequalities between social classes in incidence of disease, mortality rates and life expectancy. Doctors, then, are to be held responsible for these inequalities to the extent that it is deemed in their power to reduce them. After all, offering a reward to someone to do something makes no sense if he cannot actually do it—unless the *real* purpose of offering the reward is to manufacture a smoke screen for those who bear more responsibility and want to shift the blame onto someone else.

Are health *inequalities* in themselves *inequitable*, that is to say, unfair? As between individuals the answer must be no, unless (absurdly) fairness is demanded, ontologically as it were, of the entire universe—as if the universe had an obligation of fairness toward all the sentient beings within it. The fact is that we are *born* with different propensities to disease, and no doctor could fail to have been struck by the difference in the burdens of disease borne by different people through no fault (or virtue) of their own. A neighbor of mine has a son, now forty years old, who has suffered from Crohn's disease since the age of sixteen. He has had innumerable admissions to hospital and operations to save his life; it has deeply affected his life and career. Was it equitable (in the sense of the word used in the second article) that he alone of the family should suffer this horrid disease? Surely it is a form of inequality. It is also unfair in the sense that he certainly did nothing to deserve it; indeed, he could not have contracted Crohn's disease by actively trying to do so. Here is an instance of pure and undiluted victimhood, of an undeserved ill fate. The universe promises neither fairness nor equality.

But the differences between the health trajectories of individuals are almost certainly *not* what the article means by "disparities" that are to be reduced. Rather, it means the differences between the outcomes of various recognizable groups of humans, such as those distinguished by class, sex or race—the classification of human beings that currently obsesses not only sociologists and ideologists, but also (I think it fair to say) almost anyone who thinks about the distribution of harms and benefits in human societies. Are disparities necessarily inequitable?

There are some groups, defined by common genetic traits, that are susceptible to diseases from which other groups are immune, or almost immune. Sickle cell disease is an obvious example, or Tay-Sachs. Those who suffer inheritable diseases have done nothing to deserve them, and this is so even where the behavior of the group to which they belong increases their incidence of genetic disorders. For instance, people of Pakistani descent in Britain have a high prevalence of first-cousin marriage and therefore of inherited diseases. Should social customs be forbidden on the grounds that they increase "health inequity" as understood in the second article?

Another example of behavior with health consequences found more in certain groups than in others is that of smoking. Epidemiologists have said that the difference in the rate of smoking between the highest and lowest economic deciles in the British population accounts for half of the difference in life expectancy. (The precise proportion is unimportant for the argument, because everyone agrees that it is substantial.) Does this mean that smoking by the bottom decile should be prohibited, or that doctors should be made responsible for reducing the rate of smoking in that decile?

Sociologists would no doubt argue that a relatively high prevalence of smoking in the lowest economic decile must have a reason, such as an absence of other gratifications, or the harsh conditions of existence. But this is to deny agency to the individuals in that decile, as though they lacked any power to choose whether or not to smoke. It may be, then, that inequity in the sense of *inequality* is the price of humanity.

This idea accords with surprising statistics that I found while preparing a lecture for coroners on medicine in prison, where of course human agency is kept under tight restriction. I discovered that the standardized mortality ratio of prisoners in Britain is 1.5, which means that prisoners are 50 percent more likely to die than the general population of the same age and sex; but the standardized mortality ratio of the social class from which prisoners are overwhelmingly drawn is 2.84.[1] This means that a prisoner in England is just over half as likely to die in prison as he would be if he were at liberty to pursue his life as usual. Indeed, the life-saving effect of imprisonment is probably even greater than this, inasmuch as the prisoners were probably drawn largely from the lowest decile of the lowest decile.

At first I was shocked by these statistics, but on reflection they were perfectly plausible in the light of my experience as a prison doctor. Prison was often the only place in which some people received medical attention, not because it was unavailable to them otherwise but because they did not avail themselves of it. Outside prison they were careless as to diet and often took drugs or drank too much. All of them smoked. Thus they entered prison looking like the victims of a concentration camp and within three months were restored to good, and even strapping, health. After release, alas, they would often resume their old ways, and when they returned to prison in the same deplorable state I would say to them, "For you, freedom is a concentration camp." Although they were always said to be of low intelligence and poorly educated, the prisoners at once understood what I meant, and readily agreed.

Does this mean that we should imprison the poorest tenth of the population in the name of *health equity*, as meant in the second article in the *Journal?* ▣

---

1 The standardized mortality ratio is defined as the ratio between the observed number of deaths in a study population and the number of deaths that would be expected on the basis of the age- and sex-specific rates in a standard population and the age and sex distribution of the study population.

February 16, 2017

S ince the year 2000, more than twice as many Americans have died of overdoses of opiates and opioid poisoning than were killed in all military actions since the end of the Second World War. In 2017 alone it was over 49,000. In 2014, four times as many died of opioid poisoning as died of AIDS. Strangely enough, though, most of the Americans of my acquaintance know almost nothing of this hecatomb; perhaps it is because the deaths occur mainly among a class of person with whom they have little contact.

An article this week draws attention to a rising danger: the adulteration of street drugs with fentanyl, a synthetic opioid that is cheap to make and many times more powerful than morphine or heroin. The article does not mention that, like almost everything else these days, it is largely manufactured in China. Dealers in heroin adulterate (if that is quite the word) their heroin with fentanyl because its price per kilo is only one-thirteenth that of heroin. But those who take the heroin do not know this is done, so they unwittingly take quantities of a drug that is many times more potent and more dangerous than their usual poison, and many die of it.

What is to be done? The authors of the article draw a distinction between harm prevention and harm reduction. The former involves reducing the total amount of drugs taken in a population; the latter means reducing the harm they do once they are taken. According to the authors, these two aims may be contradictory, since a total reduction in sales would increase the dealers' motivation to "adulterate" their drugs.

(And indeed, in Britain the overall number of deaths from opioid poisoning has gone up while overall consumption of opioids has gone down.)

The authors do not ask the philosophical question whether the state is my brother's keeper—whether it is the state's business to protect people from the consequences of their free choice to indulge in drugs. With the exception of consistent libertarians, no one asks this question, and I am not sure that I would have the courage, in practice, to ask it myself.

The article suggests that one possible way of reducing deaths from opioid poisoning, and in particular from fentanyl poisoning, would be to provide those who are now (in weasely fashion) called *users* with naloxone, the antidote to opioid poisoning. Who would pay for it? That is not spelled out, but the implication is that the drug should be provided at public expense.[1]

A moral purist might say that if a man can afford to buy his own heroin (laced with fentanyl), he can afford to buy his own naloxone. If he fails to do so, therefore, assuming that he is not completely ignorant, it must be because he does not value his own safety very highly; and if he does not value his own safety very highly, why should anyone else value it more highly? He would probably be the first to complain that his rights were being infringed if the public authorities forced him to do something he did not want to do, on the grounds that he was a free citizen, fully entitled to the normal protections against arbitrary interference with his life. Why, then, should he be treated as a minor when it comes to buying a cheap product that would save his own life?

The authors conclude with words that, so to speak, bite no philosophical bullets: "We believe a full package of prevention, treatment, and harm-reduction interventions is the best bet for reducing a frightening public health threat and saving lives." And I have little doubt that, my philosophical scruples notwithstanding, I would, if I were in charge, follow their prescription, couched as it is in modern Polonius-style prose.

---

1 A purely economic argument could no doubt be produced for this. The costs of a death from opioids are not negligible. These costs are not so much in the form of lost production, as *users* are seldom among the most productive members of society. But when there is a death, there must be a police and forensic investigation, which is expensive. Naloxone is cheap.

〜

A second article attempts to tackle the question of how far the medical profession is responsible for the "epidemic" of opioid deaths. For the fact is that the American medical profession, or a portion of it, has been grossly irresponsible in its prescription of opioids. At least this has proved one thing that should have been obvious: that the harms done by drugs are not solely attributable to their illegality, but to the properties of drugs themselves when taken improperly

The authors divided emergency physicians into quartiles, according to their propensity to prescribe opioids for their Medicare (or Medicaid and Medicare dually eligible) patients who were not already taking them. They then followed up the patients of the physicians with the highest and the lowest propensity to prescribe, in order to find what proportion of them had become dependent on opioids a year later.

The doctors varied greatly in their propensity to prescribe opioids, by a factor of more than three. What the authors found was that the patients of the high-prescribing doctors were 1.3 times as likely to become dependent on opioids as those of the low-prescribing doctors. Furthermore, there was a dose-response relationship between the prescribing habits of the doctor initially seen in the emergency room and the subsequent chance of the patient developing dependence. Of course, the importance of this finding depends on the similarity of the patients seen by the high- and low-prescribing physicians.

So far, so good. But how much difference does the increased dependency rate make, in numbers of people affected? Assuming that the relationship between the prescribing habits of the doctors and the subsequent development of dependence in their patients is causative, how many additional patients did the high prescribers render dependent? If the 161,951 patients in the study who were seen by high-prescribing doctors had been seen by low-prescribing doctors, 566 would *not* have become dependent; and if the 215,658 patients who saw the low-prescribing doctors had seen the high-prescribing ones instead, an additional 759 of them would have become dependent: that is to say, about 3,250 instead of 2,500. The authors propose no mechanism by which a single visit to a prescribing emergency physician can lead to prolonged dependence, but it is not difficult to imagine one. A patient is given the impression by the physician that an opioid is the solution to his problem (and indeed he may feel euphoric after first trying it), so he seeks a continuing prescription. This may occur in only one in a hundred cases, but there are humans who are capable of grasping the wrong end of any stick, especially when it suits them to do so.

It is worth noting that even the low-prescribing doctors prescribed opioids for 7 percent of their patients. There are no data on their reasons for prescription, but I suspect that even 7 percent is far too high a proportion from a strictly pharmacological point of view. It is perfectly possible that most or even *all* patients who subsequently became dependent were started down the slippery slope by the emergency physicians, because we do not know how many of them would have done so without such an initial prescription.

Let us look at the question from the other end of the telescope. How many of the (now) millions of Americans who are addicted to opioids became addicted via high-prescribing emergency doctors? This paper does not help us answer that question, but the findings make it at least probable, and I think likely, that bad prescribing by primary care physicians may be responsible for the growth of the problem as a whole. After all, if a single encounter with an emergency room physician can lead to dependence, a more prolonged relationship with a primary care physician, who is likely to prescribe opioids a second, third, *nth* time if he prescribes them once, can *a fortiori* lead to dependence. The part played by the American medical profession in this sad story has been inglorious, even where the doctors have not been corrupt (as some of them, apparently, have been).

If doctors have been responsible for letting the genie of addiction to opioids out of the bottle, are individual patients exonerated from all responsibility for their condition or situation? I do not see that it follows. To say that they are not responsible is to say that people are not responsible for their actions unless they are insulated from any circumstances whatsoever that could have had an influence on their decisions. But this does not describe any possible human predicament. We cannot escape all influences on our choices, but we must choose, and influence upon us is not destiny. ▪

February 23, 2017

Whether or not the state has any right or duty to control what psychoactive drugs its citizens choose to consume is a matter of considerable ideological dispute. What can hardly be doubted, however, is that when things go wrong as a result of citizens' choice of what psychoactive drugs to consume, the state will be held ultimately responsible for undoing the harm done.

This much is clear from the title of an article in this week's edition: "Recreational Cannabis—Minimizing the Health Risks from Legalization." People in America increasingly have the legal (and no doubt soon to be inalienable) right to smoke cannabis, and the government has the duty to ensure that the harms caused by the exercise of that right are as slight as possible.

With commendable candor, the authors of the article say that "we should be skeptical of people who claim to know [in advance of all experience] what the net effects of cannabis legalization on public health will be." I have myself on occasion been one of those people of whom we should be skeptical, for I have prognosticated with a moral certainty far greater than any knowledge I could have had. Starting from the conclusion that I wanted to reach—that it would be wrong to legalize the consumption of cannabis—I arrived at the premises from which such a conclusion could be reached. My opponents in discussion proceeded in exactly the same manner, though of course from a precisely opposite starting point that masqueraded as a conclusion.

Legalization is by no means a straightforward concept. Does it mean that people will henceforth be permitted to buy and possess small quantities of cannabis for their personal use; to grow it but not to market it; to market it in small but not large quantities; to grow it as if it were just another crop, so that agribusiness will eventually take over and sell it like any other commodity? Will there be price and quality control, for example to limit the cannabinoid content of the plant, which is what determines its potency? In 2000, as the article points out, the cannabinoid content of an average joint was 5 percent, but selective plant breeding has increased it to 15 percent. The adverse psychiatric effects—such as paranoia—are more frequent with higher concentrations of cannabinoids.

It is not yet known whether legalization, however defined, would result in the replacement of other drugs of abuse by cannabis, or even whether it would increase consumption in the long term. The authors do point out that legalization (if of a very liberal kind) could greatly reduce the price of cannabis:

> Legalizing cannabis can dramatically reduce production and distribution costs for at least three reasons: suppliers no longer have to be compensated for the risk of seizure and arrest; it allows producers to take advantage of economies of scale; and it makes it easier to incorporate new technologies into the production process.

It is generally agreed that price has an effect on consumption: the lower the price, the higher the consumption. Demand for drugs is not, of course, *infinitely* elastic. I once worked in an environment where alcohol was virtually free, and only 20 percent of the people working there became alcoholic. Likewise, even if cannabis were available free of charge, not *everyone* would take it. Still, a low price would probably encourage consumption (especially when extra-economic costs such as illegality and social stigma have been removed), and the authors suggest ways that this result might be prevented:

> Jurisdictions seeking to ensure that cannabis retail prices don't drop precipitously have many options. For example, they could limit production, impose costly regulations on suppliers, require a minimum

price, or levy an excise tax. . . . Policymakers can learn important lessons about prevention from research on alcohol and tobacco.

I am not absolutely convinced that the analogy between cannabis on the one hand, and alcohol and tobacco on the other, is near enough for these lessons to be valuable. Cannabis is a lot easier to produce than either alcohol or tobacco. Even if the price of alcohol were to rise considerably, not many people would take to fermentation and the still; not until it became prohibitively high.[1] But cannabis being easy to produce, a smaller rise in price would provide a significant incentive to produce it. Any attempt to suppress such production would (or perhaps I should say *might*) then lead to the very situation that legalization was intended to prevent, namely, clumsy or oppressive efforts at law enforcement. The article mentions proposals to tax cannabis according to its cannabinoid content (as alcoholic beverages are taxed according to their alcohol content), but this suffers from the same objection, and it would require a considerable regulatory apparatus.

The authors say that "Since no one knows the best way to tax or regulate cannabis, creating flexible rules would make it easier to make midcourse corrections and incorporate new research and other insights into policies." This shows a rather touching faith in the way that policy is made; but the assumption behind it is that the state has a legitimate interest in regulating levels of consumption. Once this is admitted, the consistent libertarian argument for legalization is undermined. The argument for legalization becomes a purely pragmatic one, which, however, includes the fact that cannabis evidently gives pleasure to millions, and (other things being equal) pleasure ought not to be curtailed by the state without good reason.

Are the reasons for curtailment good? That will rather depend on the actual results of legalization, in whatever form legalization takes. In Colorado, it seems, various kinds of marijuana-related problems have increased since legalization, such as the proportion of fatal road accidents in which the driver had marijuana in his blood. But for a variety of technical reasons it is impossible to state that a fatal road accident was *caused* by the marijuana detected in the blood, however suggestive the

---

1 Except, perhaps, in Russia.

concentration might be. Moreover, because of Hume's dictum (which I assume to be correct) that it is impossible to derive a moral judgment from a statement of fact, it would always be possible for partisans of legalization to say that the increase in freedom as a result of legalization more than outweighed the harms done by that increase. No one doubts, for example, that people should be free to indulge in team sports, even though they may—in fact they *do*—result in many avoidable injuries. If it is argued that the participants voluntarily accept the risks involved in sport (assuming they know what the risks are), the fact nevertheless is that such injuries impose costs on others, at least where medical assistance depends on third-party insurance. Bringing home *all* the costs of risks to those who take them is impossible, as impossible as any utopian dream, and would besides turn many of us into extremely timid beings afraid to do anything much. The point at which we forbid certain types of risk taking depends on judgment and not just on scientific information. Bismarck said that the whole of the Balkans was not worth the bones of one Pomeranian grenadier. Are the pleasures of a million dope smokers worth the death of one extra person in a road accident? I do not see a way of answering that question beyond all possible dispute; but it would be common sense that they would not be worth the deaths of a hundred thousand extra deaths in road accidents.

The authors do not reflect upon the question whether a man *ought* to intoxicate himself. Again, it rather depends on how frequently he does it, in what circumstances, and what form his intoxication takes. Voluntary intoxication is no defense to a crime, and indeed many people (including Aristotle) view it as an aggravating circumstance rather than a mitigating one. On the other hand, intoxication adds greatly to the gaiety of humanity, including—in its milder forms, with alcohol—to my own.

I have long suspected that underlying the debate about the legalization of cannabis is the question whether the search for personal pleasure, self-indulgence if you like, is or ought to be the highest goal of mankind and of individual men. At the risk of sounding puritanical (a risk for which I *do* accept all the consequences), I will say that I think it is not, and moreover it is usually self-defeating. But the connections between law, morality and the proper ends of life are complex, and it is possible for reasonable people to disagree about them. I accept that my instinctive feeling that the loosening of controls on cannabis is likely to be harmful and culturally retrogressive might be wrong. ◙

March 2, 2017

Genetic engineering has not so far kept its promise, at least in its most optimistic, not to say utopian, form. There has been no sudden extension of human life expectancy or decline in the chronic diseases to which heredity contributes, only the same steady improvement that has been going on for so long that we have come to think of it as being in the natural order of things. But, as my financial adviser never tires of telling me, past performance—presumably including poor performance—is no guide to future performance. Perhaps the genetic nirvana is just around the corner, if time has corners.

A paper in this week's *Journal* brings the goal of gene therapy a little closer. A team of doctors and researchers in France seem to have cured a child of his sickle cell anemia, at least temporarily. Before his gene therapy at age thirteen, he had 1.6 sickle cell crises per year and treatment with regular transfusions; in the fifteen months since the therapy, he had no crises and no need of transfusions. Moreover, his red blood cells were now much closer to normal in their physiology.

I cannot pretend to understand the technical procedures of the treatment, but in essence the team replaced the boy's red blood cor-puscle–forming cells with genetically altered cells, the alteration being introduced via a harmless virus. How long the beneficial effect will last, or whether the procedure has any long-term deleterious effects, cannot yet be known; presumably it will be reported later.

There are other caveats also: sickle cell anemia is a relatively straightforward genetic disease in which the replacement of a single molecule of the DNA causes a deficient variant of hemoglobin to be produced. In fact, it was the first such disease to be fully elucidated biochemically. Most diseases to which heredity makes a contribution are not so straightforwardly genetic in origin. Usually there is more than one gene involved in the disease's transmission and development, and environmental factors also play a much bigger role.

Moreover, the expense of this treatment must have been enormous (though it is not given in the paper). Even allowing for the tendency of techniques to become cheaper as they become routine, it is difficult to imagine how this technique could ever be cheap enough to be applied to all the people suffering from the disease. If that is so, one can foresee ethical problems looming in the future. Assuming that funds for health care remain limited, access to the treatment will have to be rationed, *de facto* or *de jure*. Who should be offered the treatment, and who not? There is ample opportunity for the development of conflict, and this is all the more so when the principal sufferers from the disease are black.

An article about the history of sickle cell disease in the same issue of the *Journal* gives a foretaste, or an intimation, of what might be to come (including conflicts over rationing of treatment if it remains very expensive). Those who suffer from the disease are most unlucky. They are subject to repeated infections and extremely painful crises in the course of which they may suffer strokes and destruction of bones. They suffer from profound anemia. Their growth is adversely affected, and often their intellectual development is too. Their life span is much reduced, though it has risen dramatically since 1910, when it was about two or three years, to about fifteen years when I qualified in 1974, and now to nearly forty-five years. But that is still much below a normal life span, and even that foreshortened life is filled with much suffering.

The improvement achieved to this point was brought about by the use of antibiotics and blood transfusions, and latterly by hydroxyurea, for the treatment of infections, reduction of anemia and promotion of the production of healthier red blood cells. None of these is the magic bullet that is the cynosure of so much research effort. Gene therapy is the first magic bullet for sickle cell disease.

In order for someone to develop sickle cell disease, both parents must have one copy of the defective DNA that causes it. The parents are then said to have the sickling trait, though not the disease itself, or only a very mild form of it under extreme physiological conditions, for example when there is less oxygen in the air. But a quarter of the children born to parents both of whom have the trait will have the full disease.

Sickle cell anemia is often used as an explanatory example of Darwinian theory. Why has a defective form of DNA survived quite extensively in a population when those who are homozygous for it— having two copies of it in their genetic material—have such a reduced life expectancy under natural conditions that they do not reach the age of reproduction? The answer is that those with the sickling trait are more resistant to malaria, and the populations among which the defective DNA is found originated in areas of the world in which malaria, itself often fatal at a very early age, is prevalent. Overall, then, the defective DNA conferred a survival advantage on those who possessed it; in certain circumstances it was not defective. The question then becomes one of why the *entire* population did not have it.

In other circumstances, of course, the defective DNA confers no advantage. Once it was possible to recognize the sickling trait in blood, it should in theory have been possible to eliminate the disease by genetic counseling of would-be parents (assuming that they all followed the counsel given). But as the article on the history of the disease notes, "aggressive counseling of couples with sickle cell trait to avoid having children ran into accusations of racial genocide." Such accusations are absurd. At most, 10 percent of American blacks have the trait, so the genocidally inclined would hardly have chosen this method.

Hyperbole, however, is the stock-in-trade of identity politics, and increasingly of all politics. The great chemist and biochemist Linus Pauling no doubt helped to fuel it:

> Pauling contributed to the controversy by suggesting that "there should be tattooed on the forehead of every young person a symbol showing possession of the sickle-cell gene or whatever other similar gene…[because] if this were done, two young people…would recognize this situation at first sight, and would refrain from falling in love with one another."

Pauling may have been a great biochemist, but (if this is any indica-tion) he knew little of the human soul, whatever the moral status of his proposal. People often fall in love despite rather than because of ratio-nal calculation; indeed, I have known people to fall in love, or at least indulge in sexual congress, because of the particular danger involved. For example, I had a patient who used the fact that he was positive for human immunodeficiency virus as a means of attracting sexual partners.

But let us just suppose for a moment that Pauling's proposal would be effective, *grosso modo*, and that the numbers of children with sickle cell disease would be greatly reduced as a result of the compulsory tattooing of people to indicate the bearing of the gene for it. What is actually wrong with the proposal, then? Would not the tangible ben-efits—diminished suffering, heartbreak and expense—greatly outweigh harms done by it? After all, no one could suppose that bearing the trait was a moral defect meriting persecution or even mere mockery. If you should reply that this is to forget how much persecution and mockery people have endured in the past for abnormalities that were none of their fault, we respond: "But we are more enlightened now."

I do not know how to answer the question other than by my general revulsion against the involuntary branding of human beings. (That so many of them now seem eager to brand themselves with tattoos hardly answers the case.) If someone were to reply that he felt no such revul-sion, and that for him tangible good always weighed more heavily than intangible harm, I would not know what to say to him.

There is another interesting little lesson to be drawn from the article. In 1972, President Nixon, reacting to a perceived and perhaps real lack of research into the disease, signed the Sickle Cell Anemia Act allocating money for such research. Alas, "Even Nixon's promise of funding proved divisive when it became clear that without congres-sional appropriations...the money for research on sickle cell disease was diverted from cardiovascular research." Where there is competition for resources, you cannot discriminate in favor of something without discriminating against something else. ∎

March 9, 2017

In his "Ode on a Distant Prospect of Eton College," the melancholy poet, Thomas Gray, questions whether apprehension of the future increases or destroys happiness, and he ends with two of the most famous lines in English poetry—so famous, in fact, that most people do not know whence they come. Speaking of the pupils of Eton College playing happily in the mid-eighteenth century, Gray says:

> Yet ah! why should they know their fate?
> Since sorrow never comes too late,
>   And happiness too swiftly flies.
> Thought would destroy their paradise.
> No more; where ignorance is bliss,
>   'Tis folly to be wise.

Maybe so, but then the question becomes one of knowing when ignorance is bliss. This requires some insight into what the effects of knowledge would be in any individual case. Ignorance can also be agonizing.

An article titled "Anesthesia and Developing Brains—Implications of the FDA Warning" draws attention to the potentially harmful effect of the precautionary principle: the principle according to which something is to be avoided or prohibited because of the potential and plausible but unproven harms that it might cause.

On December 14, 2016, the FDA (Food and Drug Administration) issued a "Drug Safety Communication" to the effect that general anesthesia and sedative drugs used in the treatment either of pregnant women in the last three months of their pregnancy or of children in the first three years of their life "may affect the development of children's brains." Needless to say, this created some alarm, as well as surprise, for such communications are supposed to be based upon the best scientific evidence possible. Most doctors do not have the time to look into the evidence themselves and come to a reasoned conclusion, so they have to rely on someone's authority in making their decision. If doctors had to investigate the truth claims behind everything they did, medicine would soon be rendered completely impotent and every doctor would be a Hamlet.

According to the article, the "communication" was based upon inadequate evidence. This is not quite the same as saying that it was wrong: evidence might still emerge that proved it correct. Knowledge is always finite, while ignorance is always infinite.

The evidence upon which the FDA relied for its warning was that the exposure of a variety of animals, or animals' neurons, to sedatives or anesthetic agents had "immediate neuroanatomical consequences and associated long-lasting ... functional effects." The species of animals in which the effects were found ranged from roundworms to primates. But man is not a chimpanzee, let alone a roundworm, nor were the situations of their exposure even analogous to those of the exposure of mothers and children to the agents concerned. It is dangerous to argue that if something happens in situation *a*, it must happen in situation *b* with some passing resemblance to it. In medicine, it is not a question of what *should* happen, but of what actually does happen.

The evidence of what actually happens is often difficult to interpret, however. It is true that long-term adverse neurodevelopmental effects have been observed in young children who have been exposed to prolonged or repeated anesthesia, but of course those children were suffering from serious or life-threatening conditions that themselves affected, or might have affected, neurodevelopment, such as chronic lack of oxygen in congenital heart disease. In these cases, there was no alternative to operation under anesthesia, other than continued illness and probable death. The choice in medicine, as in politics, is not often between perfection and catastrophe, but more commonly between different evils.

Insofar as there is relevant evidence about the effect of a single short exposure of infants *in utero* or in their first three years of life to an anesthetic, it is reassuring. The question has been investigated in the General Anesthesia vs. Spinal Anesthesia (GAS) trial and in the Pediatric Anesthesia and Neurodevelopment Assessment (PANDA) trial. (Controlled trials in medicine are now often given an acronymic title that aids memory, and sometimes I have wondered whether the science follows the acronym rather than the other way round: whether someone has thought up a splendid acronymic name for a trial, and then performs it.) The GAS and PANDA trials found no neurodevelopmental effects of single short episodes of anesthesia, for example in caesarean section. The results do not apply to longer or repeated anesthetics, but as we have seen, such anesthetics are not given to children who would otherwise be neurodevelopmentally normal.

The warning given by the FDA, then, is premature and unfounded. But the FDA is supposed to be some kind of clearinghouse for medical research, sifting the evidence to find what is and is not safe, like a Supreme Court of patient safety, and so its animadversions have been attended to. Quite large numbers of cases are involved: each year at the Texas Children's Hospital alone, 13,000 children under the age of three are anesthetized, 1,300 of them for more than three hours. Of the latter 1,300 cases, two-thirds are for congenital heart disease. In no cases can surgery be postponed until the brain is thought to be less susceptible to damage. (Incidentally, there is no reason why three years should be a cut-off point for concern: the human brain continues to develop well after that age, even if conduct sometimes doesn't appear to do so.) As the authors of the article point out,

> Indicated procedures in pregnant women and young children that can safely be delayed are rare.[1] Until reassuring new information from well-designed clinical trials is available, we are concerned that the FDA warning will cause delays for necessary surgical and diagnostic procedures, resulting in adverse outcomes for patients.

In other words, the FDA has stirred up anxiety for no very good reason—even if it might subsequently be proved that anxiety was justified.

---

1 This may not be true in the case of caesarean section, whose rates vary quite widely according to factors other than the danger to mother or child.

Meanwhile, the Texas Children's Hospital, in response to the FDA communication,

> has adopted the warning's recommendation that a discussion occur among parents, surgeons and other physicians, and anesthesiologists about the duration of anesthesia, any plan for multiple general anesthetics, and the possibility that the procedure could be delayed until after 3 years of age....

The problem is that these discussions will inevitably "occur" in conditions of considerable ignorance, an ignorance that almost certainly will persist for years if not decades to come, given the great difficulty in answering some of the scientific questions involved: for example, whether delaying an operation until after the age of three really does avoid neurodevelopmental harms, and whether those harms must be offset against other harms caused by delay in operation, including a decreased rate of survival.

It is often necessary to act in the absence of full information, and anxiety can be raised to no good purpose. To adapt slightly Thomas Gray's lines: "Where ignorance of ignorance is bliss, 'tis folly to be wise."

I hope I shall not be accused of cynicism, however, when I say that I perceived a little cloud forming on the horizon thanks to the FDA's warning: the prospect of civil lawsuits. How long before some grieving parent sues on the basis of that warning? In a litigious society, whatever happens is grist to the lawyers' mill.

An elderly lady of my acquaintance has been kept alive well beyond her life expectancy at the time she was diagnosed with chronic myeloid leukemia by a drug called imatinib. A paper in the *Journal* showed that the effectiveness of this drug did not decrease with time, and in effect it cured a condition that previously was fatal. The death rate from the disease in the United States and elsewhere has been halved, probably as a result of the introduction of the drug.[2]

---

2 With all due caution against the common mistaken argument of *post hoc ergo propter hoc.*

Imatinib was discovered and developed by Novartis, the vast Swiss pharmaceutical company. The general image of drug companies is that they are nothing but predators upon the sick or upon health-care systems. Here is a case that casts doubt upon that easy assumption. Of course, it is still possible for the enemies of drug companies to claim that imatinib could just as well have been discovered by some other organization, such as a government laboratory. Nevertheless, the fact remains that it wasn't; and that it *was* developed by the *ex officio* evil Novartis company. ◼

March 16, 2017

Individual case histories are not much in favor in medical journals these days, although the *NEJM* carries one a week taken from the records of clinical-pathological conferences held at the Massachusetts General Hospital. These cases are usually of rare or complex diseases, and I for one am always astonished that the doctors seem always to get the cases right, at least as to diagnosis if not as to outcome. A high proportion of the cases result in death, despite all the ingenuity and erudition expended upon them.

In this issue there is also a different kind of case history, used to make an emotional appeal for a change in policy. It is titled "Another Senseless Death—The Case for Supervised Injection Facilities," and recounts the story of someone called Frankie. It begins:

> Frankie liked to tell people that "we made our bones together." He must have said that a hundred times, to every new medical student I introduced to him, to every nurse, and during every one of our many visits. I had a general sense of what he meant, but on the morning that I heard that he's died of an overdose the previous night, I finally looked it up. Popularized by *The Godfather*, the expression has come to mean taking action to establish respect.... That Frankie's favorite phrase started as a criminal reference and evolved into a pathway to respect seems fitting, a metaphor for his life.

As is so often the way these days, the word *respect* is here used with a special meaning, conflating the sense it has in "I respect your right to your opinion" with that in "I respect your opinion." Those are two very different things, in fact. I respect your *right to believe* that the Pacific Ocean is made of chicken soup, but I do not respect your *belief* that it is made of chicken soup.

In the modern urban sense, *respect* means fear, either physical or moral. The person who demands rather than earns respect in this sense intimidates his interlocutor. In this case, Frankie demands that the author pass no moral judgment on the way he has chosen to live, and not express the opinion that it is wrong or degrading, for that would be lacking in *respect*. His sanction against her (the author is a woman) would be to withdraw cooperation from her, and as a compassionate and conscientious doctor she would be hurt by this. Compassion these days means accepting without demur someone else's point of view, rather than keeping in mind that it is wrong but also that we are all miserable sinners, so to speak, and there but for the grace of God go I.

Frankie, it turns out, was an injecting heroin addict who "had been incarcerated for more periods than he'd been free." Significantly, the author does not tell us what he'd been in prison *for*, perhaps because the information might have reduced our *respect* for him somewhat. It is possible that he had been in prison for minor offenses, but also possible that he had been in prison for violent offenses (such as street robbery) that caused a lot of misery to others. He certainly caused a great deal of misery to his ancient mother, whose husband and other son also died of overdoses.

Implicitly (I think) we are supposed to feel sorry for Frankie because his life of imprisonment and reimprisonment is to be regarded as a misfortune, in the way that suffering from a chronic neurological disease would have been, even though there is no allegation that he suffered any injustice. But in fact, imprisonment may well have been a benefit received by Frankie rather than a wrong or harm done to him, because we learn that "his periods of injection-heroin use had been interrupted only by his prison terms." (The word *abuse* is avoided, for that would be stigmatizing.) Thus he might well have died sooner if he had not been incarcerated, just as he might have survived if he had been incarcerated for longer.

This certainly accords with my experience working as a prison doctor in England (though I admit that my experience might not be readily transferable across the Atlantic). Heroin-addicted offenders would arrive looking almost moribund but then would quickly regain their health in prison. As I have mentioned, the standardized mortality ratio of prisoners, by comparison with that of the social class from which they are mostly drawn, indicated that being in prison substantially reduced their risk of dying. This is a sad commentary on our society, and certainly on the human condition of these, our fellow men.

As for Frankie, it was not that no effort was made to save his life once he was out of prison. The author of the article cared for him for seven years and "there was probably no patient I worried about more," she writes. Heroin, we learn,

> gave him a few hours of respite. It gave him relief from the memories of being locked in a cage; from the worry about being 50 with no ability to get a job or find housing because of his criminal record and no skills other than ones that were sure to land him back in prison; from the flashbacks to finding his brother, and then his girlfriend, dead from an overdose; from the guilt over the pain he knew he caused his 85-year-old-mother.

We are here implicitly being asked to believe that Frankie took heroin to alleviate his problems, rather than that his problems were caused by his taking heroin. It is true, of course, that once he had taken heroin for long enough, his existential situation was unenviable: it would indeed have been difficult for him to pick up as if he were an adolescent or young man at the outset of his career. Fifty is not the age at which one begins anew; and his suffering was no doubt real enough. But we should not pretend that it was other than self-inflicted even if we decide that it is useless or counterproductive, after so many years, to confront him with the fact.

The author, however, is not addressing Frankie in her article. She is addressing doctors, and she should not varnish the most evident truth by pretending that being a victim of your own behavior is no different, morally, from being a victim of circumstance or of other people's conduct. One does not become an injecting heroin addict by chance or overnight. Most such addicts have taken heroin intermittently for some time—many months—before they become addicted. They have to accommodate themselves to its unpleasant side effects; they all know beforehand what heroin addiction entails; they have to learn such things as how to obtain heroin, how to prepare it, how to inject it (and probably to overcome an instinctive reluctance to inject themselves). Heroin addiction is not something that happens to a person; it is something that he consciously *wants*. It is a perverted desire, but it is still a desire.

Frankie was prescribed medication and was sent to rehabilitation (all at other people's expense, of course). None of it kept him off the heroin for more than a few weeks. The author thinks that he would have survived if there had been a facility to which he could have gone where he injected himself with heroin in the presence of professionals, who would have revived him in case of overdose. There are such facilities in other places, and they do appear to save addicts' lives. Whether Frankie would have used one had it been in existence cannot be known for certain.

But does such an expedient constitute medical treatment? Is it very different, morally, from giving habitual robbers large sums of money to desist from their robbery? Almost certainly it would be found to "work," except perhaps for those "addicted" to the excitement of robbery. I suspect also that it would not encourage many people to become robbers, for I am still sufficiently starry-eyed about human nature to believe that it is not only because of a fear of the consequences that we refrain from robbing others on the street.

In her final peroration, the author says that the establishment of a facility for addicts to inject themselves safely would be an "important step," one that "recognizes that people who use drugs have not forfeited their human rights, including the right to safety and health." One could write a book on the confusions and misconceptions in this passage. Suffice it to say that no one infringed my human rights when I fell ill, nor is the fact that I am mortal an infringement of my rights. It is a condition of being alive at all. ▣

March 23, 2017

In 1977, R. D. Rosen coined the term *psychobabble* and characterized it as follows:

> a set of repetitive verbal formalities that kills off the very spontaneity, candour, and understanding it pretends to promote. It's an idiom that reduces psychological insight to a collection of standardized observations that provides a frozen lexicon to deal with an infinite variety of problems.

It was clever of Rosen to have spotted, named and described something that was to become an enduring, even growing, part of social life. Much later, I said that psychobabble was the means by which people could talk about themselves without revealing anything.

Psychobabble is now a seemingly ineradicable part of our culture, and one of the first *NEJM* articles this week is full of it. The article is titled "Breaking the Stigma—A Physician's Perspective on Self-Care and Recovery." The title assumes, of course, that stigma must be harmful in itself and that it can play no positive part in our social existence. No one could doubt that stigmatization can be unfeeling, cruel and unthinking; to blame a child for being illegitimate, for example, is to blame it for the conditions of its own conception. This is absurd as well as cruel, but it was common for much of our history.

However, this is a far cry from showing that stigma and stigmatization are always to be reprehended. I think many of us would behave worse than we actually do were it not for fear of stigma; and this fear cannot exert its effect unless stigma itself exists, at least as a possibility. It is true that fear of stigma can drive you to commit evil along with people bent on evil; but by the same token it can impel you to do good, if not to be good. A society in which nothing is stigmatized (if such a society were genuinely possible) would be a society without standards.

The article in the *Journal* begins in confessional mode:

> My name is Adam. I am a human being, a husband, a father, a pediatric palliative care physician, and an associate residency director. I have a history of depression and suicidal ideation and am a recovering alcoholic....I am a survivor of an ongoing national epidemic of neglect of physicians' mental health.

Even here there is an important evasion. Many people who drink too much often claim to be depressed. A few people drink too much when and because they are depressed in the true, but now rarely used, sense of the word. Of those who drink too much and are depressed, however, the great majority are depressed because they drink, for alcohol in excess is a depressant. This is an important distinction. But those who are depressed because they drink too much are implicitly claiming to have an illness that makes them drink, and that therefore they are not responsible for intemperate behavior.

Fortunately, the author is now "recovering." (He understandably doesn't say "recovered," any more than an ill-tempered man can say that he has finally conquered his temper.) His amelioration, if not his cure, has been brought about through "counseling, meditation and mindfulness activities, exercise, deep breathing and hot showers." I have nothing against exercise or hot showers (and in fact I take at least one hot shower a day myself), but they hardly seem to fall into quite the same therapeutic category as antibiotics, say, or anticancer drugs. If it is replied that they alter brain chemistry, this is presumably true of all human activity, from opening the refrigerator to reading the newspaper. On this criterion everything is either illness or therapy, or both.

The author's "confession" that he is a human being, a husband, a father, etc., actually tells us very little about him. It is like the answer that a late (and much-lamented) Australian judge of my acquaintance gave a man who asked him what kind of car he had, trying thereby to place him on the socioeconomic scale. Having no interest in cars himself, the judge replied, "A green one," which is about as individualizing as is the author's description of himself.

Having informed us of his therapeutic methods, the author continues: "I've worked hard to develop self-awareness—to know and acknowledge my own emotions and triggers—and I've set my own boundaries in both medicine and my personal life." This is precisely what Rosen called psychobabble, the "idiom that reduces psychological insight to a collection of standardized observations that provides a frozen lexicon." It is abstraction piled on abstraction.

"I learned that I must take care of myself before I can care for anyone else," the author tells us. If I were to ask you to go and find someone who had learned to care for himself before he looked after someone else, who or what would you look for? It might, indeed, be someone in the Ayn Randian mold, a person who believes that selfishness is not only permissible but actually the highest and only virtue. At any rate, you would have no very clear idea at the outset of your quest.

The need to look after himself being the first lesson the author learned, the second was "about stereotyping," which of course is always wrong. The author says he has learned to be "intolerant" of stereotypes. "Alcoholics are stereotyped as deadbeats or bums," he writes, which I think is far from the truth. I think most people, certainly most readers of the *NEJM*, have a much more nuanced notion of alcoholics than the author allows, and are fully aware that alcoholics are to be found in almost every stratum of society. They do not think all alcoholics are of the homeless type who sleep over air vents of buildings to keep warm in the winter. Moreover, no words could be more stereotyping than *deadbeats* or *bums*, but surely we do not have to be told that people are individuals with unique life stories even while falling into types. I cannot now recall a time when I did not know this. But in any case, what would a person be like if he had *no* stereotypes in his mind whatever? He would be as defenseless as a newborn mouse.

There is a strange combination of high-mindedness and special pleading in what the author writes:

> Mental health and substance-abuse conditions have no preju-
> dice.... When you live with such a condition, you're made to feel
> afraid, ashamed, different, and guilty. Those feelings remove us further
> from human connection and empathy.

But are not fear, shame, difference and guilt universal human qualities? If they removed us from human connection and empathy, then human connection and empathy would never be possible. Moreover, fear, shame and guilt are often justified; and an alcoholic who has ruined his family's life for years is rightly ashamed. A lack of such shame would be shameless, and shamelessness is far from an admirable quality. In effect, the author is making a plea for his own innocence, because he assumes what is false: that a man who is even partially to blame for his own situation is unworthy of compassion. This is certainly not the Christian view, nor is it (I would say) that of anybody who thought about or reflected on man's position in the world.

Another lesson that the author learned, though not necessarily a good one, is that "being honest with myself about my own vulnerability has helped me develop self-compassion and understanding." Here psychobabble meets Uriah Heep. "Be vulnerable, Uriah, be vulnerable." Self-compassion here sounds remarkably like self-pity, and few are the people so lacking in compassion that they fail to feel sorry for themselves. The author's notion of being honest with himself almost amounts to a plea for *dishonesty* and a permanent evasion of the duty of self-examination. It is a manifestation of the *true-me* psychology, according to which there is an immaculate inner core of myself that is so good that it need never—indeed, *must* never—feel any fear, shame or guilt.

What we have in this article is a self-portrait without a portrait. I think you could go to a dinner party with the author, or even take a holiday with him for a month, without realizing that he was the author of this supposedly confessional piece. Of course, it might be said that the article does no harm: except, I would say, that no one will answer it (or, if he does, will not have his reply published), so that its assertions and general tenor will go by default. We shall continue to live in a world of emotional slush. ▣

March 30, 2017

There is nothing quite like having a disease, or being at risk of developing that disease, to encourage one to read articles about it in medical journals. Like most men of my age (though after what I have just written, I don't want to sound confessional), I suffer, or at least experience, symptoms of an enlarged prostate. I have had two friendly acquaintances who died of cancer of the prostate, which is one cause of such enlargement, and one of them died at my present age. I was therefore more than commonly interested to read a review article titled "Prostate Cancer Screening—A Perspective on the Current State of the Evidence." It may actually have changed my life.

As everyone thinks he knows, prevention is better than cure, but this principle is, in the case of screening, bedeviled by many caveats. And the whole question of screening for prostate cancer is formidably complex to answer, perhaps even unanswerable.

The screening procedure itself is straightforward: a regular blood test to detect levels of prostate-specific antigen (PSA). A rapidly rising level is supposed to indicate cancerous growth. So far, so simple.

But even here, without further ado, there are questions to be asked: How often, and at what ages, should the test be performed? Every year? Every two years? Between the ages of sixty and seventy-five, or at some other period in life? Experiments to answer these questions would be difficult to perform, their interpretation would probably be contentious, and in any case (given the immense time and cost involved) they will probably never be done.

According to the authors, the best guess, or guesstimate, of lives saved by PSA screening is one per 1,000 persons screened in ten or fifteen years. This unimpressive figure would not matter so much if screening had no adverse effects, if it did only good and no harm, but this is definitely not the case. The problem is that the more screening is done, the more false positive cases are found. Moreover, cancer of the prostate is often an indolent disease, progressing very slowly and causing no symptoms or suffering, which means that even a correct diagnosis might be of no benefit. But once cancer has been diagnosed on the basis of heightened PSA, hark what discord follows!

The person diagnosed with such cancer naturally begins to feel anxious, whereas before he was not anxious. This is only a minor problem, however, compared with others. When a man is diagnosed with cancer of the prostate, he is likely to undergo biopsy of the prostate, removal of the prostate or radiotherapy of the prostate. These procedures are not without complications. For example, those who have undergone prostatectomy have a 20 percent higher rate of incontinence and a 30 percent higher rate of impotence. Radiation treatment is associated with a 17 percent higher rate of impotence and also problems with bowel function.

Nor is this all. While the problems associated with interventions are immediate, the benefits (if any, which is far from certain) are in the quite distant future, from the patient's perspective. The life is saved not immediately, but in several years' time. How many years of incontinence, in how many patients, are worth the value of one life saved? There is no unambiguous way of measuring this.

The finding of cancer where there is none, or of cancer so indolent that it will not affect the patient's life, has become so commonplace as to create a so-called epidemic of prostate cancer. In the United States, screening came to be very widely performed, no doubt for commercial reasons, *before* its effects were known, or before any proper experiments had been done. And once people have come to believe that screening is advisable, it is more difficult to find controls for properly conducted experiments. After all, who will volunteer to forgo a procedure that he believes might well save his life?

In 1988, at what the authors call "the dawn of the PSA era," the incidence of prostate cancer was estimated at 135 per 100,000. By five years later it had risen to 220 per 100,000, a 63 percent increase. Then, as the blind faith in PSA screening declined, so did the rates of cancer: by 2009, the incidence had fallen back to 150 per 100,000. These changes of incidence were probably caused by changes in the rate of testing, not in the disease itself.

These statistics mean that when screening was most heavily promoted, seven men in 10,000 screened had cancer wrongly or unnecessarily diagnosed. Factor in the estimated rate of lives saved by screening, and it would mean, further, that many men had cancer wrongly diagnosed for every life saved (supposing that any lives at all were saved). Thus, for any individual, the chances of PSA screening doing him harm are much higher than the chances of it doing him good, albeit that the good (saving his life) is a very considerable one—assuming that saving him from cancer of the prostate is not merely making him available to death by some other cause at the same point in life. Cancer of the prostate is a disease of comparatively late age, when men are more likely to die from any number of causes. The article mentions only cancer-specific death rates, not all-cause death rates, and this omission is very important.

The article on the whole is admirably clear, but it makes a highly ambiguous statement to the effect that there has been a "decline of approximately 45% in U.S. prostate cancer mortality from the late 1980s to the present." Does this mean that 45 percent fewer of the *population* at risk are dying of the disease, or that 45 percent fewer of those diagnosed with the disease are dying of it? I think the former is probably meant; but in either case, the fall is probably not due to screening, because treatment of cancer of the prostate during that period has improved. Any screening program whose efficacy is measured by the death rate over a prolonged period from the disease screened for is trying to hit a moving target: if treatment of the disease has improved during that time, then any decline in the death rate may be wholly attributable to better treatment rather than to screening. In fact, the death rate from prostate cancer is declining along with the decline in screening, but this does not by itself prove that screening is ineffective, since it is at least conceivable that the death rate might have declined further if screening had continued at its previous rate.

It seems to me that all these difficulties with PSA screening are unlikely ever to be met, and certainly not in my lifetime. In fact, the following authorities have advised against PSA testing at any age: the U.S. Preventive Services Task Force, the Canadian Task Force on Preventive Health Care, the American College of Preventive Medicine, and the American College of Family Medicine. Granted, the argument from authority is not an argument at all: it is not as if the history of human authority were one of uninterrupted progress toward Truth. Still, those recommendations collectively are probably not without significance. Even the American Urological Association, which might have been thought to have a vested interest in PSA screening, gives only a qualified recommendation:

> Implement shared decision making for men 55 to 69 years of age and proceed on the basis of men's values and preferences, recommend against screening for other ages.

The American College of Physicians recommends something similar:

> Discuss benefits and harms for men between 50 and 69 years of age and order screening only if clear preference is expressed for screening; recommend against screening for other ages.

In other words, let the men decide for themselves after an examination of the evidence.

Even raising the possibility of screening is not a neutral act without consequences, however. Some men will ever afterward wonder, and worry, whether they have made the right choice. They are being asked to decide in the context outlined at the very beginning of the article:

> After a quarter century of extensive screening for prostate cancer with prostate-specific antigen (PSA) in the United States, and after the completion of two major trials examining the effects of such screening, the medical community is still divided with regard to its effectiveness and its benefits-to-harms ratio.

And the poor patient has to make up his mind after a ten- or fifteen-minute consultation!

Suffice it to say that I will not be screened for prostate cancer, at least not with my knowledge and consent, though the real reason for my refusal is not that I read this article. It is just that I don't want to be. ◼

April 6, 2017

"**I** was only obeying orders." These seemingly simple words have had a sinister ring to them ever since they were used by functionaries of the Final Solution in an attempt at self-exculpation. No one who had done something good would be likely to say that he was only obeying orders in so doing.

But in fact all of us were only obeying orders for much of our lives, and many of us, perhaps, do so for our entire lives. This is inevitable, at least in a highly complex society such as ours. There must be authority of one kind or another, even if we want as little over us as possible. When we fly, we are pleased that the captain is in control, even if, very, very occasionally, the captain turns out to be incompetent, wicked or suicidal.

Early in their careers, all doctors obey orders. They have to do so and, on the whole, trust the system that has put their seniors over them, to guide and educate them until they in their turn become seniors. Fortunately, there has always been a consensus on how doctors should comport themselves and how they should act.

As the powers and prowess of medicine increase, however, previously unimagined ethical dilemmas arise. Moreover, with reforms in society, what was previously thought to be unethical becomes ethical, and vice versa. In Britain, for example, attempting suicide was long a crime, and when someone tried to shoot, gas, poison or hang himself, the doctor had a duty to report it to the police. This would now be regarded as not only cruel, but a flagrant breach of confidentiality. In the old days, once the person had recovered from whatever it was that he had done to himself, he was charged with a crime. When the law was abrogated, the numbers of attempted suicides exploded.

Changes in the law may clash with some doctors' deep-held ethical or religious beliefs, such as on abortion. If the law permits it, must the doctor perform it, or act as an accessory, perhaps by advising a patient who wants an abortion where she may procure it? At what point may the doctor refuse to go along with the prevailing wisdom?

This question is posed in an article titled "Physicians, Not Conscripts—Conscientious Objection in Health Care." It draws a parallel—only to refute it later—between a doctor refusing a certain kind of treatment and a conscript refusing to fight in a war that he believes to be wrong. The first paragraph runs:

> "Conscience clause" legislation has proliferated in recent years, extending the legal rights of health care professionals to cite their personal moral beliefs as a reason to opt out of performing specific procedures or caring for particular patients. Physicians can refuse to perform abortions or in vitro fertilization. Nurses can refuse to aid in end-of-life care. Pharmacists can refuse to fill prescriptions for contraception. Recent state legislation allows counselors and therapists to refuse to treat lesbian, gay, bisexual, and transgender (LGBT) patients, and a recent lawsuit seeks to excuse states from providing gender reassignment surgery and other health care services to transgender patients.

I don't think you would have to be Sherlock Holmes to guess in which ethical direction this article will eventually lead. There is a small clue, by means of euphemism, in the sentence "Nurses can refuse to aid in end-of-life care." What is clearly meant here is that nurses are allowed to refuse to kill their terminally ill patients. And since the article concludes that "it is incumbent on professional societies to affirm professional role morality and authoritatively articulate the professional ethical standards to which all licensed health care professionals must adhere," it is easy to deduce that where euthanasia or physician-assisted suicide is permitted, sanctioned and practiced, nurses not only may but *must* kill their patients when instructed to do so. But what if the ethical worm turns, and suddenly it is decided that euthanasia and physician-assisted suicide are really murder after all: will the nurses who killed their patients despite their misgivings be able to fall back on the argument that they were only obeying orders?

The problem is a complex one, of course, and I suspect that it is yet another situation in which judgment rather than law is required. It is obvious that doctors cannot refuse to treat their patients on bizarre ethical grounds; there has to be *some* ethical consensus. For example, it would be very wrong to refuse to treat a transsexual for pneumonia, but refusing to perform transsexual surgery is a very different matter. Allowing people to make up their own code of ethics according to their entirely personal precepts would be wrong; but enforcing every last rule would likewise be wrong.

The article argues that "the proliferation of conscientious objection legislation in health care violates the central tenet of professional role morality in the field of medicine: the patient comes first." But what is right for the patient may not be what the patient wants. He may not want what he actually needs, and he may desire what he does not need. The doctor is enjoined to do what he thinks is best for the patient, not carry out his wishes in all circumstances.

A case in point is the rather peculiar person who cannot feel sexually satisfied while he has his full complement of limbs, and therefore wants one leg amputated to achieve fulfilment. He may tell the surgeon that if he, the surgeon, does not carry out the amputation, he will do it himself, perhaps by sitting with one leg over the railway track as a train goes by. At least one surgeon has succumbed to this moral blackmail and I do not think he should have done so; but at the same time I do not believe that he should be hauled up before some kangaroo court for a breach of ethics. And if you approve of transsexual surgery, on what reasonable grounds could you say that what he did was wrong?

The authors of the article, who are *health ethicists*, say that a professional medical association should be the arbiter of a doctor's conduct and, collectively, the profession's conscience, and in general this is so. But shortly after I read the article, I read elsewhere that there is a proposed law before the Dutch parliament that would extend the right of euthanasia, carried out by doctors, to elderly people who, though not terminally ill, were tired of life and thought their productive, useful, happy lives were at an end.

Now if ever there was a slippery slope begging to be slid down, this is it, for one may be tired of life at any age. Indeed, adolescent angst and Weltschmerz is by no means uncommon. And who is the doctor to decide whether such *taedium vitae* is genuine or not, or whether it is sufficiently long-lasting for him to kill the person who says that he suffers from it?

If a person has a right to euthanasia, moreover, someone must have a corresponding duty to carry it out. Unless a special group of people is trained for the purpose, that someone will be a doctor or a nurse. (The existence of a specially trained group of killers, the euthanasians, would be chilling. Imagine a child in school being asked what he wanted to be when he grew up and he replied that he wanted to be a euthanasian.)

Once it has been decided that killing people who are tired of life is permissible, and furthermore that they have a right to easeful death, it will become the duty of doctors to kill, and this will become an accepted clause of the code of medical ethics. For, as the article in the *Journal* puts it, "The health care professional who wants to prioritize personal values over professional duties must choose a less personally fraught occupation."

I don't have an answer to the difficult question of how far and in what circumstances individual doctors may be allowed to decide ethical matters for themselves. I doubt that there is a doctrinal answer that will meet all cases, without exception. But the *NEJM* article has an unpleasantly totalitarian ring to it: for according to the authors, all doctors *must* act in compliance with precisely the same code of ethics once the official body of the profession has laid it down, and must change their conduct when the official body tells them to. ◼

April 13, 2017

The great poet Alexander Pope wrote of "This long disease, my life," and he did not mean it metaphorically: he had chronic Pott's disease, tuberculosis of the spine, which gradually crippled him. But no one, least of all Pope himself, would have wished that he had never lived, or called his life meaningless. Health is obviously desirable, but not the only desideratum of life, and even very bad health does not render life worthless. Today, however, health is thought so important that whatever promotes it is deemed to be permissible or even obligatory, and whatever harms it to be reprehensible or prohibited.

Sport is often touted as health-giving, as if this were a sufficient justification and even a necessary one. But sporting activity is not the same thing as sports events, with a small number of participants and large numbers of spectators. Are such events good for a society's health? An article in the *Journal* examines how the general population might be affected by marathon races, which have relatively large numbers of participants, but they are not the focus of the study; rather it is the overall effect of the events themselves on survival from heart attack.

The authors analyze the death rate of persons who have heart attacks on days in which marathons are run in big cities in America. Their hypothesis is that the road closures made necessary by the marathons delay ambulances in reaching patients and taking them to hospital, thus delaying their treatment and increasing mortality from heart attacks. They analyzed data from 121 marathons, in eleven cities, from 2002 to 2012, looking at death rates in the thirty days following a heart attack that occurred on marathon days, and comparing those with death rates following heart attacks on the same day of the week in the five weeks before and the five weeks after the marathon.

In short, the authors found that the death rate following heart attacks on marathon days was 3.3 percent higher than that following heart attacks on other days. Among the latter, 24.9 percent of the patients died within thirty days, but for marathon-day heart attacks the figure was 28.2 percent.

The increased deaths were not caused by heart attacks occurring among participants in the races. The authors cleverly reanalyzed the data including only those patients who were very old and had five preexisting medical conditions, and who were therefore most unlikely to have participated in the marathons. The difference in death rates persisted. Moreover, the difference did not appear among those heart attack patients who lived just outside the marathon area and were taken to different hospitals.

On average, the running of the marathons led to a delay of 4.4 minutes in hospitalization, from 13.7 minutes to 18.3 minutes. Although other explanations for the rise in death rates cannot be altogether ruled out, the authors conclude: "Our findings are consistent with the idea that delays in care attributable to infrastructure disruptions are a possible explanation."

Let us for a moment accept the hypothesis in its strongest form: that the additional number of deaths was wholly attributable to delays caused by road closures: how many people, in absolute numbers, died as a consequence? According to the statistics given, 1,145 heart attacks occurred on marathon days, of which 323 led to death. On nonmarathon days, 11,074 heart attacks occurred, of which 2,757 led to death. If the rate of death from marathon-day heart attacks had been the same as from heart attacks on nonmarathon days, 38 fewer people would have died (which is slightly less than one person for every three marathons, though the paper does not include this analysis). Of course, because of statistical uncertainty, it might have been more, but by the same token it might have been less.

Could this small increase in death caused by marathons be justified by the personal gratification of the thousands of runners who participate? I do not see how there can be a definitive answer to this question other than some kind of global but not indisputable judgment. One death is the extinction of a universe, so to speak, and we are enjoined to think of every human life as infinitely precious. But we can hardly think this in reality, or we would not permit any risk to life at all. Some risks are worth taking, others not. Here the risk is to a third party who has not himself agreed to take it, which complicates the matter. But the risk is very tiny in comparison with the numbers supposedly put at risk, who theoretically might have a heart attack on a marathon day. There is no discussion of the seriousness of the risk in the paper, which in fact suffers from a very common defect of papers that measure risks: giving only relative and not absolute risks. If, on reading such a paper, you have to work out the absolute risk for yourself, the chances are that whatever has been found is not very important. If it had been important, the authors would have trumpeted it.

Moreover, increased risks can sometimes be outweighed by reductions in other risks. A paper in the *British Medical Journal* some years ago suggested that heart attacks among marathon runners—which, incidentally, occurred predominantly in the last mile, so going the extra mile is precisely the most dangerous thing to do—were more than compensated for by the reduction in fatal road accidents that would have occurred if the roads had not been closed.

For myself, the running of a marathon recently brought an unexpected benefit. I arrived in Geneva on the day of the marathon there, and the man who invited me could therefore not pick me up at the airport in his car. I took the train instead, which was much quicker.

We are all prone to conspiracy theories, perhaps for biological reasons. "Why should Mr. Y. trust non-Diné medicine and doctors?" asks a physician who works in primary care among Navajo Indians on a reservation. (Apparently, Diné is now considered a more correct name for the Navajo.) The doctor's article in this week's *NEJM*, titled "Lessons from Standing Rock—Of Water, Racism, and Solidarity," suggests that his patient's mistrust is understandable given the historical dispossession of Indians. In other words, Mr. Y.'s racism should be condoned, and perhaps even applauded.

Mr. Y. suffers from Type 2 diabetes. There has been a marked increase of late in the prevalence of Type 2 diabetes among his ethnic group. The author continues: "Why would he not consider the ugly possibility that the very system that may have caused his diabetes now benefits by entangling him in a web of demands to maintain his health?" This is a very weaselly way of putting it. The question "Why would he not...?" teeters between psychology and logic, without ever quite partaking of either or choosing between the two, so it is immune from criticism.

The reason why Mr. Y. should not consider the ugly possibility is that it would not be intellectually correct to do so, except on the supposition that all white men are the same, all equally disposed to evil (which he presumably does not believe, or else he wouldn't have consulted the doctor in the first place). He almost certainly has Type 2 diabetes because he has a genetic predisposition and, more importantly, he is overweight through having consumed too much of a very poor diet, possibly promoted by advertising but still consumed by him. If his health is to improve, he will have to do what everyone else with the disease has to do: eat differently.

The *Journal* for April 13 also carries two research articles and an editorial about Type 2 diabetes. The editorial is titled "Increase in the Incidence of Diabetes and Its Implications," and it begins:

> Diabetes mellitus is among the most prevalent and morbid chronic diseases, affecting the health of millions of persons worldwide. According to the Global Burden of Disease report for 2015, the prevalence of diabetes rose from approximately 333 million persons in 2005 to approximately 435 million in 2015, an increase of 30.6%.

In the United States, the incidence of Type 2 diabetes rose 4.8 percent a year during the same period, though fastest among nonwhite ethnic groups. If this rapid rise is the result of a "system," it must be a pretty large and well-directed system, a little like the Judeo-Masonic communist finance-capital system beloved of...oh well, best not to say.

The well-meaning doctor on the Navajo reservation asks in his article, "In a history marked by cultural domination, how do I uphold my pledge to 'do no harm'?" I think the first thing might be to discourage conspiracy theories. ◼

April 20, 2017

It has often been claimed that the harm done by illicit drugs is very largely, if not entirely, caused by their illicit status. If only they were freely available, any harm they do would be negligible, a small price to pay for the increase in personal liberty that free availability would represent. But the current epidemic of deaths from opioid overdoses in the United States, which by the end of 2017 had killed more than 300,000 persons, suggests that this is a rather simple-minded view. No one applies the same principle to the harms done by cigarettes.

An editorial in the *Journal* is titled "Addressing the Opioid Epidemic—Opportunities in the Postmarketing Setting." One would not expect incisive prose to follow such a title, as indeed it does not. Very near the beginning, however, is an implicit recognition that the epidemic represents a startling failure of the regulatory system:

> The preapproval evaluation of drugs is meant to ensure that they are safe and effective for their intended use. Nevertheless, widespread use of approved drugs often leads to identification of safety issues, including rare adverse events that may not be detected in preapproval trials...and a small percentage of drugs are withdrawn from the market.

This is a slippery formulation, designed to exculpate the relevant authorities. What happened, in fact, was that oral opioid drugs were deemed by those authorities to be safe and appropriate treatment for patients with chronic pain (such as backache) because it had been shown that vanishingly few patients given strong painkillers for acute or cancer pain ever became addicted to them in the sense that they either craved, sought out or further took the strong painkillers once the acute pain ended. From this was extrapolated the absurd idea that such drugs would be perfectly safe for use by those with chronic pain.

I do not think that any practicing doctor with a minimum of clinical experience would have failed to note the differences between patients with acute or cancer pain, and those with chronic pain. It is true that among people with acute pain there are differences related to temperament, age, culture and so forth; but with chronic pain the very large component of psychological "overlay" (as doctors often disparagingly call it) is much more evident. In fact, the physiology of the two categories of pain is very different, and research has shown that the intensity of chronic pain is not proportional to the pathology by which it is occasioned. It correlates closely with the sufferer's sociopsychological condition, whereas acute pain does not. One man with acute gout may scream, while another only grimaces and holds on to himself, not uttering a sound; but no one doubts that both suffer from severe acute pain.

So the very basis on which opioids were licensed for use in chronic pain was flawed, to put it mildly. There was, of course, a history to the loosening of controls on prescription: for many years (I remember them well), strong painkillers were denied even to those who might have benefited from them, mainly because of the fear, mistaken as we have seen, that addiction might result. Even people with but a short time to live, who were certain to die within a few weeks, were denied such painkillers, often very cruelly. The decision to loosen the opioid tap, as it were, was in part to atone for past puritanism in the matter, now seen as sadism. And so the gamekeeper turned poacher.

This is interesting in itself, for it suggests that there is no history or experience from which the wrong lesson cannot be drawn. That two wrongs do not make a right is a cliché, of course, but in our conduct we often disregard the truth it expresses. If drought is bad, it does not follow that a flood will be an unqualified good.

With the loosening of the tap, certain drug companies saw the possibility of turning a drip into a flood. They embarked upon a campaign of propaganda in favor of prescribing opioids to all and sundry who complained of pain. The article states that the efforts of Purdue Pharma included:

> hosting 40 all-expenses-paid speaker-training conferences for 5000 practitioners, as well as 20,000 pain "education" programs. Purdue used physician profiling to target high-volume opioid prescribers with sales representatives who were encouraged by a generous bonus system. Branded promotional items and free starter coupons for patients were available.

All this was perfectly legal at the time, if unscrupulous. But once the genie was out of the bottle, as it were, returning it there has proved very difficult. Not that the efforts to do so have been very great: it was only after scores of thousands had died that anyone seemed to take any notice.

The *NEJM* is not generally known for its humor, but the following raised a smile (of a kind):

> Even today, the risk-benefit profile of opioids used for chronic pain remains unknown....The harms associated with opioid use...are well-documented and often dose-dependent. They include abuse, addiction, hyperalgesia [increased pain], overdose, fracture, pneumonia, erectile dysfunction, motor vehicle crashes, cardio-vascular events and death.

As the deaths are currently running at 49,000 a year (2017), the benefits of opioid use for chronic pain would have to be very considerable indeed, almost miraculously so.

In fact, as another article in the *Journal* not long ago pointed out, there is no evidence at all that opioids are of any value whatever in the treatment of chronic pain. "A recent review identified no studies lasting longer than 1 year that evaluated pain, function, or quality of life as a primary outcome," it reported. This may be true in a literal sense, but the absence of longer studies does not mean that we cannot draw relevant inferences from the studies that have been done. It is unlikely that drugs found to be of no value in the relief of pain in the shorter term will suddenly become effective once the one-year mark is passed.

There is a clue to the reasons for the authors' somewhat muted approach to the problem of opioid addiction resulting from medical prescriptions:

> Beginning around 2010 [i.e. many years into the epidemic], our clinic made several changes to improve the risk-benefit profile for management of chronic pain [note the avoidance of the more forthright term, *harm*-benefit profile]. We adopted controlled-substances agreements, implemented urine testing and prescription-drug-monitoring programs, convened an opioid review committee to assist physicians with difficult cases, started using pharmacists to help oversee opioid prescriptions at the clinic level, and provided education, support, and access to pain-management specialists. More recently, we fully integrated medication-assisted treatment for addiction in the primary care setting, providing a crucial evidence-based tool for treating high-risk patients.

This is a virtual admission in bureaucratese that "our clinic," and others like it, bore responsibility for creating the epidemic in the first place. As for providing access to pain-management specialists, this is like offering alcoholics the keys to the brewery.

I used to watch patients headed for the pain clinic in my hospital bounding up stairways and showing no evident distress, until they reached the portals of the clinic, whereupon their pain would assume agonizing proportions. They left the clinic clutching their prescription for dangerous drugs. It seemed never to have occurred to the doctors in the clinic to observe their patients' behavior outside their consulting rooms, or even to doubt their word. The clinics appeared to need private detectives at least as much as they needed psychologists.

Doctors, of course, don't like to disbelieve their patients, and on the whole they are right not to do so. But I recall one case on which I was asked my opinion where disbelief would have been entirely proper. A young man who had been prescribed strong painkillers told his doctors repeatedly that he had lost his prescription, and they kept re-prescribing until he was taking enormous dosages per day. Then he decided to sue his doctors for negligence because of his strong addiction to the painkillers. I was asked my opinion by lawyers as to whether the doctors had been negligent. Strictly speaking, I said, they had been. But whether doctors can be blamed very much for believing the lies of their patients (in this case, preposterous ones) was a question I would leave to the courts to decide. In this case, the law acted with common sense: irrespective of the conduct of the doctors, that of the patient had been so dishonest that he deserved no compensation. The case was struck out at an early stage. ▣

April 27, 2017

I t is odd that people often take up positions according to their political or philosophical preconceptions on subjects that ought to be matters of fact. Chief among these subjects (at the moment) is that of global warming. If someone says that he is a conservative, the chances are that he will consider global warming a hoax perpetrated on the world by those who, disappointed by the triumph of capitalism over socialism, want a new pretext to rule the world. Conversely, those who want to rein in capitalism will latch on to global warming as a pretext for doing so.

Though we are told that global warming is the question of questions, I have, strangely enough, taken little interest in it, and have no firm opinions on it (not that mere ignorance precludes firm opinions). For what it is worth, I do not find the idea of global warming caused by man's activities to be as absurd as some of my more doctrinaire friends say it is. I have traveled quite a lot, and I have been struck by how much of the world's surface seems visibly covered by a grayish-pinkish-mauvish-purplish haze even on the finest day—when, in fact, it is most obviously visible. Surely this haze, or some component of it, which is clearly the work of man, traps heat? Alas, I am no physicist to give the answer.

It seems to me that there are several questions that need to be answered, and I am not qualified to answer any of them:

   1. Is global warming happening?

2. If it is, is it as a result of man's activities?
3. If it is, is carbon dioxide the principal cause?
4. Is global warming altogether a bad thing, or does it have offsetting advantages that might even outweigh its disadvantages?
5. If the harms it will cause are serious, what is the best way of averting them?

An article in this week's *Journal* titled "Preventive Medicine for the Planet and Its Peoples" outlines many of the harms caused by global warming, many of them as yet hypothetical. I confess that the notion of preventive (or any other kind of) medicine for the planet irritates me and seems to me redolent of a modern reversion to paganism, but let that pass. The article is not without its virtues, among them clarity.

The harms to health caused, or yet to be caused, by global warming are laid out:

> With warming temperatures come longer summer heat waves that increase mortality, particularly among vulnerable populations—elderly and poor people, residents of urban heat islands, and people with mental illness. Higher temperatures also increase ozone levels, compromising lung function and exacerbating asthma. Earlier and longer pollen seasons elevate exposure to allergens, increasing allergic sensitization and asthma episodes. Higher temperatures result in larger and longer forest fires, reducing downwind air quality and increasing hospitalizations for respiratory and cardiovascular conditions.
>
> Climate change is also making dry areas drier, wet areas wetter, and severe storms with heavy precipitation more common. Hurricanes and floods kill people directly, and their indirect effects, such as waterborne-disease outbreaks following floods, cause broader harms to human health. Warmer water temperatures also facilitate the growth of pathogenic waterborne organisms such as coliform and vibrio species.
>
> The distribution of vectorborne diseases such as Lyme disease, West Nile virus, Rocky Mountain spotted fever, plague and tularemia expands as the range of their vector changes. The distribution of the Lyme disease tick, *Ixodes scapularis*, for instance, is projected to

expand to cover most of the United States over the next 60 years. The mosquito vectors of pathogens not currently common in the United States, such as dengue, chikungunya, and Zika, may find more favorable conditions.

One is—or at least I am—struck by how much hypothesis and how little fact there are in that passage. This does not by itself make it wrong or mistaken, for hypotheses may be correct; but it does mean that those who deny the baleful effects of global warming, at least as far as health is concerned, cannot necessarily be dismissed as mere cranks. No effect size is mentioned or even hypothesized. There is no mention either of a paper published not long ago in the *Lancet* that analyzed an immense quantity of data regarding death rates and ambient temperature and found that lower-than-normal temperatures were associated with (one cannot say *caused*) seventeen times as many deaths as were higher-than-normal temperatures. This raises at least the *possibility*, though very far indeed from the certainty, that large areas of the globe will become more healthily habitable if global warming occurs. And while the authors of the *NEJM* article assume that global warming will disrupt rather than increase food supplies, this is questionable.

A graph that accompanies the article raises my suspicions too. It shows the mean temperature of the surface of the earth from 1880 to 2016. Certainly there has been a sharp trend upward since 1980, but there was a forty-year plateau before that, and no rise at all between 1880 and 1935. I am afraid this graph reminded me rather of those given me by my financial adviser to demonstrate just how splendid his advice has been. One cannot help but think that the dates and scales of the graph are selected to prove a point rather than to demonstrate a truth found by disinterested inquiry. Moreover, the span from 1880 to 2016 is fairly short in geological time, and surely the climate didn't begin in 1880 any more than sex (according to Larkin's poem) began in 1963.

For all that, as I look out of my window on a cloudless day and see that grayish-pinkish-mauvish-purplish haze on the horizon, I cannot help but wonder whether the climate alarmists are right.

∽

Being on the lookout for dogs that remain silent in the nighttime, I spotted one in an otherwise excellent review article about the physical abuse of children. It starts with a clinical vignette and goes on to describe how the subject of the vignette should be investigated further. The story is as follows:

> A 4-month-old male infant is brought to the emergency department by paramedics. His mother had dialed 911 because the infant appeared to be limp when she lifted him from his crib after she returned from work; she had left him with her boyfriend while she was at work.... The physical examination [of the child] is normal except for decreased muscle tone, and there is a 1-cm bruise on his left cheek.

Although the article is mainly concerned with the investigation of a child's physical signs in such a situation (such as abnormal scans, x-rays or enzyme levels), it is unusual for there to be no nod in the direction of etiology and epidemiological distribution of the condition under consideration. For example, there was a similar review article about sickle cell disease the week before, with much information of this kind in the vignette. Why the difference?

There is a clue in the narrative: "she had left him with her boyfriend while she was at work." The sad fact is that the kind of parenting that this phrase suggests is highly propitious for the physical abuse of children. The boyfriend was not the father of the child, I assume, for otherwise the mother would have been reported to have left it with his father. And considering that the child was only four months old, I think it fair to surmise that the boyfriend who caused the injury would not be the last of the mother's boyfriends. It is well known that stepfathers are much more likely to abuse children than biological fathers, especially those who are married to the mothers of their children. None of this is mentioned in the article except very elliptically, in these words: "a more extensive social history should be obtained, including who was caring for the infant during the mother's absence and whether other children were in the home." Anything more explicit might bring a blush to the cheek of those who have suggested for years that it matters not under what dispensation or arrangements parents beget children.

Here truly is a dog that did not bark. The delicacy of it and the desire not to cause unnecessary offense would be admirable in other contexts, but not in this. ◼

May 4, 2017

When we bought our house in a remote rural area, we were already fifty-five years old, an age at which health often begins to decline and medical emergencies become more common. Considerations of medical care played not the slightest part in our decision to buy the house, and did not even enter our heads as a concern. Was this foolishness or wisdom? I think there can be no definitive answer; it depends upon one's scale of values. Though access to health care may sometimes be a precondition of life, there is more to life than access to health care. Nevertheless, if ever we need emergency medical care while at our house, we are as good (or bad) as goners.

A paper from Denmark in this week's *Journal* suggests that, in the event of a cardiac arrest, we are less likely to survive, and also less likely to survive without brain damage, than if we lived in—well, Denmark. The aim was to measure the benefits of provisions for cardiac emergencies that are being made widely available in Denmark.

The authors traced the outcomes of every cardiac arrest that occurred in Denmark outside hospital over a period of twelve years, from 2001 through 2012. They analyzed the data according to whether the person affected had received no assistance from bystanders, or cardiopulmonary resuscitation or defibrillation from bystanders, or resuscitation from professional emergency medical staff sent out to assist him. Outcomes were measured in terms of the rate of anoxic brain damage and subsequent admission to a nursing home, one year after the event, in those people who had had a cardiac arrest and had survived for at least thirty days.

In the twelve years studied, there were 42,089 people in Denmark who had cardiac arrests outside hospital. Of these, 7,630 were excluded from the study because they were already suffering from anoxic brain damage or already living in a nursing home. This left 34,459 cases available for the study.

During the period of study, the rate of thirty-day survival after cardiac arrest increased from 3.9 to 12.4 percent. (Over the entire period, the rate was 6.3 percent.) This improvement the authors attributed to the increased training of the general population in cardiopulmonary resuscitation and the increased availability of automated defibrillators in public places in Denmark. By the end of the study period, not only did a higher percentage of people survive cardiac arrest by thirty days or more, but a smaller percentage of the survivors suffered brain damage or needed to be admitted to a nursing home. The rate of brain damage or admission to a nursing home for those who survived cardiac arrest by thirty days went down from 10 percent in 2001 to 7.6 percent in 2012, a highly significant statistical difference.

Yet the histogram provided in the paper prompted me to regard this way of framing the results as highly doubtful, not to say dishonest. It shows the rates of brain damage or admission to a nursing home in each individual year between the start and finish of the study, and there were several years in which the rate was higher than in the starting year. In the years 2006, 2007, 2008, and 2009, for example, the rate was higher than in 2001 (and considerably higher in 2007), while in the year 2011 it was the same.

Thus, by choosing the year 2012, the authors got the result they wanted, much in the way that financial advisers or sales representatives of pharmaceutical companies do. If the results were quite as happy as the authors suggest they were, one might have expected a more or less smooth improvement in the rates, rather than the ups and downs that actually happened. The end date of the study was therefore highly convenient: and this raises suspicions that the start date might also have been chosen with a predetermined conclusion in view.

The twelve-month death rate from any cause after cardiac arrest was certainly lower in 2012 than it was in 2001, but it was lower in 2005 and 2006 than it was in 2012. Besides, people who have cardiac arrests tend (on the whole) not to be the healthiest of people, so they may die from other incidental diseases not caused by whatever brought on their cardiac arrest. In other words, a decline in the all-cause death rate after successful resuscitation does *not* demonstrate a decline in the relevant twelve-month death rate after cardiac arrest, because there are many potential causes of death or survival.

But let us take the improving thirty-day survival rate after cardiac arrest at face value: what would it mean? If during the same period the rate of anoxic brain damage or admission to a nursing home did *not* decline, or declined at a slower rate, it would mean that the absolute numbers of people with such anoxic brain damage or living in a nursing home would actually have increased, possibly by a considerable margin. What is presented as a triumph for public health and safety would thus, at the very least, have certain costs to which the paper, either from boyish enthusiasm or a desire to cover up, does not refer.

The question, then, is a very unpleasant one: how many anoxic brain-damaged persons or persons confined to nursing homes are equal to one person saved from premature death who goes on to lead a normal life? Health economists have tried to answer this question with various scales, the most famous of which is the "quality-adjusted life-year," or QALY, but attaching a figure to an incommensurable comparison does not increase accuracy; it only gives people a false sense of assurance that their decisions are purely rational.

This paper, it seems to me, offers a *post facto* justification for decisions already taken—namely, to train everyone in cardiopulmonary resuscitation and provide defibrillators everywhere. These decisions *may* have been right or wise, and in fact most decisions have to be taken before it can be known whether they are right or wise, but this paper certainly provides no evidence one way or the other. It strikes me as more rhetoric than dispassionate science.

The authors are confident that they were able to trace almost *every* out-of-hospital cardiac arrest that occurred in the entire country during the twelve years of their study, thanks to the highly developed and efficient information system in Denmark, which gives to each of the five and a half million citizens a "unique Civil Personal Registration Number that is used in all health care contacts." This may excite the reader's admiration, or horror, or some combination of the two. It certainly increases efficiency, presumably making your entire medical history instantly available to any doctor or hospital in the country that treats you; and every doctor knows that there are few things more frustrating and time-consuming than not having access to a patient's previous medical records. And yet, at the same time, there is something a little nightmarish about a system that, in principle, knows everything about you, over which you have no control, and that you are powerless to alter. Danes no doubt trust their state, and perhaps (so far) they have every reason to do so, but we who live in less favored lands do not have quite the same confidence in our masters.

The authors say that rates of cardiac arrest remained constant in Denmark over the study period, yet one of the principal causes of cardiac arrest, coronary artery disease, has been in sharp decline over the past decades, and one might therefore have expected the rate of cardiac arrest to decline as well. That it did not would suggest an increased propensity to diagnose cardiac arrest in conjunction with a decrease in actual cardiac arrest, but the authors do not sufficiently consider the possibility that this might explain an improvement in rates of thirty-day survival after a supposed cardiac arrest. If the real rate of cardiac arrest declined while the rate of people surviving alleged cardiac arrests increased, we are in the presence not of triumph but of farce.

At any rate, the paper teaches one valuable lesson: that it is necessary to pore over such a publication in order to detect its true meaning, if any. The notion that a scientific paper, at least in medicine, yields up its meaning at a glance is false. But we often give such papers only a glance. ▪

May 11, 2017

It was with a sinking heart that I picked up the *Journal* this week, the title of its first article legible through its transparent plastic wrapper: "The Future of Transgender Coverage." By *coverage* was meant insurance coverage, not media coverage; it referred to the means by which things that some people need or want should be paid for by other people.

A statistic in the article caught my eye: 0.6 percent of adult Americans are "transgender," which amounts to 1.4 million persons in all. This is given as a definite figure, as if it were a fact in the same way as that there are fifty states in the Union. But what do we find when we turn to the *Diagnostic and Statistical Manual of the American Psychiatric Association* in its fifth and latest edition? This publication is not exactly reluctant to give high prevalence rates of all the conditions that it enumerates: for example, it quotes a figure (that only psychiatrists in search of patients could fail to laugh at) of 1.5 percent for the so-called "dissociative identity disorder," formerly known as "multiple personality disorder." What prevalence does it give for what it calls "gender dysphoria"? It suggests 0.005 to 0.014 percent of males and 0.002 to 0.003 percent of females. On the assumption that there are roughly as many men as women in the population, and using the maximum rather than the minimum figures provided, we find that the prevalence is 0.0085 percent.

Now the *DSM*, as it is known for short, was published in 2013, hardly an eon ago. What happened in the intervening four years that led to a seventyfold increase in the prevalence? There are, of course, epidemics of infectious diseases with even more startling increases in prevalence than this; but it seems to me that if you wanted to know what was going on, you would be better advised to study the vagaries of fashion than look for something comparable to an outbreak of typhus.

Curiously enough, though the *NEJM* article makes reference to the *DSM*, it does not mention the discrepancy in prevalence rates, as if it were of no interest or possible significance. Here is another dog that refrained from barking.

I looked up the problem of people changing sexes in a textbook dated 1979, called *Sexual Deviation*, edited by Ismond Rosen. It was probably the most authoritative text on the subject of its time, and though thirty-eight years is (or at least once was) not a long time in the history of a civilization, the book has the air of having been written in a different epoch. For one thing, the very word *deviation* in its title would now scarcely be used, it is so inherently *judgmental*; and for another, there is a fustiness to it that might just as well be Victorian or Edwardian. It starts with the statement: "In recent years there has been a resurgence of interest in sexual behaviour." I confess that I laughed. Was it the interest itself in sexual behavior, or the way in which the interest was expressed, that had changed?

In 1979, *transgender* was not even a word; the term used was *transsexual*. Actually, the word *transgender* is for once probably more appropriate: for while sex is a biological matter, gender refers to social and behavioral traits that are generally, but not always, aligned with sex. Be this as it may, the book makes statements that today would result in the social ostracism of the author, if not (in the more socially advanced legal jurisdictions) lead to outright arrest. For instance:

> Male transsexualism is an oddity, then, not only because the condition is so strange—a male who tries to change into a female—but for reasons of interest to those concerned with psychodynamic theory. This is especially true of the oedipal development in the transsexual boy....[1] In treating adult male-transsexuals, the general rule has

---

1 Interestingly, the existence of the Oedipus complex is here taken to be as indubitably factual as the date of the Battle of Hastings. Is there a law of the conservation of dubious assumptions?

been that whatever one does, it is wrong.... While the ideal would be a masculine man, it is hard to see how that can occur in a person who has never had any masculinity built into his personality from infancy.

Gender dysphoria is in essence a strange, not to say bizarre, feeling and desire. According to the *NEJM* article, "every major expert medical association in the United States" recognizes the medical necessity of assuaging and satisfying this desire by means of "transition-related care." This, of course, is the argument from consensus and authority, and it would not be difficult to find past consensus or authoritative statements from medical associations that would now strike us as wrong or even evil.

How far is the satisfaction of feelings and desires in such matters to go? Odd as transsexualism may have struck the author of the chapter in Rosen's book, there are odder sexual deviations yet: for example, apotemnophilia and acrotomophilia (which are not included in Rosen's book). The first of these is the desire to be an amputee in order to find sexual fulfilment, while the second is the finding of sexual fulfilment only with an amputee. Despite valiant attempts to ascribe these peculiarities to neurological dysfunctions, none has been found. They are just as much disorders, or abnormities, of feeling and desire as is transsexualism.

The arguments for the *medical* necessity of enabling the transsexual to *transition* (as the ugly contemporary locution puts it) are just as strong for the apotemnophiliac. An amputation of a perfectly healthy limb, though unnecessary by normal medical criteria, is no more disfiguring than sex-change operations and hormonal treatment, nor is it more irreversible. Should the apotemnophiliac change his mind, artificial legs are very good these days. As for any social disadvantages that might result, legislation could be enacted forbidding, say, football teams from discriminating against those who have had amputations for such purposes. There could even be Apotemnophilia Pride parades, thus killing two birds with one stone: fulfilling the population's desire to demonstrate its broadmindedness in public, and satisfying humanity's eternal prurience. The only regrettable absence, given the state of art teaching in the West, is that there would be no Daumier to record it.

The *NEJM* article says, "Transgender people's need for care that affirms their true selves and promotes their health and well-being parallels all Americans' desire for high-quality, affordable health insurance coverage and health-care." Let us overlook the possibility that many Americans may have no such desire; in a large population, there are all types of people. Instead, the concept of *affirming the true self* bears, and indeed requires, some examination.

Behind the *ex cathedra* statement of the article's author, who hails from the Johns Hopkins School of Public Health, are several assumptions: that the true self is a kind of fixed entity independent of one's will, behavior and habit; that the true self, whatever it is, must essentially be good and therefore worth expressing; that it is the purpose of medical care to allow people to express that self; that a person's true self *ought* to be affirmed, even if his true self is like that of Jeffery Dahmer. All of this seems to me to be very doubtful, to say the least. Even supposing that the true self can be found, distinct from all other selves such as the purely phenomenal one (the self that is apparent to observers), is it the job or purpose of medical care to affirm it, or the responsibility of others to pay for the affirmation? The article makes the point that impoverished transsexuals of socioeconomically disadvantaged groups have particular difficulties in making the "transition" for financial reasons. In essence, it pleads for their treatment to be paid for by others.

Before I be written off as a monster of insensitivity, let me admit that there seem always to have been people uncomfortable with their biological sex, and add that I think that there are sometimes good reasons for plastic surgery to be carried out for aesthetic reasons. People may be born with or acquire deformities or disfigurations that understandably make them miserable; and the division between these and minor anomalies that offend pure vanity may not always be clear. But this is another matter entirely. ▪

May 18, 2017

A doctor, I suppose, should be interested in everything human—in every ill to which flesh is heir; but it is only human also to be more interested in those subjects with which one has some direct connection than in subjects utterly remote from one's personal experience. Two articles this week aroused in me important memories of my own past, the first concerning asthma, and the second, acute heart failure. When I was fifteen a close friend of mine, a year older than I, died in an acute asthma attack. When I was about twenty-six, I suffered acute heart failure, as a result of a disease from which the death rate was between a quarter and a half.

My friend who died of asthma was taking by inhaler a drug, isoprenaline, that relieved his symptoms but put a strain on his heart and was later found to increase the death rate in asthma. He was also taking what was then a new drug, sodium cromoglycate, to prevent certain cells in the lung, called mast cells, from bursting during an allergic reaction and releasing various substances that cause the bronchi to constrict and thereby make breathing difficult, labored and finally (in his case, alas) impossible. I shall never forget the day that I learned of his death. He was an intellectually brilliant young man whose life, though short, had been long on suffering. Severely eczematous as well as asthmatic, his entire body was covered in little scales that he shed everywhere, and his chest was deeply deformed by the damage done to his lungs from birth.

All this was more than fifty years ago, so I was both interested and sad to read a trial of another drug, imatinib, which inhibits an enzyme that provokes the production of mast cells, in cases of refractory asthma, which is asthma that does not respond well to normal treatment. An editorial points out that mast cells, which are found in everyone, can't be all bad, because "evolution has not endowed us with mast cells to fill our asthma clinics or to permit us to develop allergic disorders," and that therefore their total elimination cannot be altogether desirable. Reducing their number in those who suffer from their oversensitivity would be a good thing, but it might prove difficult to get the balance right.

The small controlled trial of imatinib (31 patients given active treatment, 31 given placebo) showed that the drug substantially reduced the reactivity of the airways of asthmatic patients. This is a hopeful result, though the authors are cautious enough to warn that "the data are not clinically directive," by which they mean that it is far too early to recommend the routine prescription of imatinib. "It is possible," they write, "that the effect we found with regard to airway hyperresponsiveness will not translate into a clinical benefit in larger studies."

If I were subsequently to read of imatinib's great success in treating refractory asthma such as that of my friend, what would my feelings be? They ought, of course, to be those of undiluted pleasure because so much suffering would be relieved; but in practice I think they might be somewhat more ambiguous. I might, unreasonably, feel a slight bitterness that my close friend (who I am sure would have made a valuable contribution to the world of scholarship and was very modest despite his brilliance) did not live to receive the benefit of it. Why should he have suffered and died when those like him today survive and are relieved of their suffering? This may not be unjust, but it is very unfair.

A much larger trial of a new vasodilating drug called ularitide, to be used in acute heart failure, was a resounding and definitive failure. More than 2,000 patients with acute heart failure were assigned either to ularitide by intravenous injection or to placebo. Of the patients given ularitide, 236 died; of those given placebo, 225 died. This was not a statistically significant difference; ularitide was neither better nor worse than placebo. It had been hoped that the swift treatment of heart failure with a vasodilating drug would improve the prognosis; but as an accompanying editorial puts it, the trial of ularitide "lessens the likelihood that there is a constructive avenue for the further development of natriuretic [sodium secreting] peptides." It also squashes the idea, at least for the moment, that there should be rapid-response teams dedicated to treating people with acute cardiac failure such as I had forty years ago. In my case, nature took its course, which, fortunately for me, was benign. There seems to be nothing at the moment that alters the outcome in this situation.

There were a couple of sentences in the editorial that I had some difficulty in construing:

> At this point, we should remind ourselves that the primary immediate objective of treatment is the patient-centric goal of symptom relief....This conclusion will allow us to change the focus from disease modification so that mortality is once again relegated to a safety, not an efficacy end point.

If I have understood correctly (which is not certain), this means we should give up trying to save patients' lives and merely make them comfortable.

∽

There was a famous book in the 1950s of the title *Only in America*, and I could not help thinking of it as I read an article titled "Physicians, Firearms, and Free Speech—Overturning Florida's Firearm-Safety Gag Rule." Apparently the Florida legislature had passed a law forbidding doctors from "routinely entering any information on firearm ownership into patient records, discriminating against patients on the basis of firearm ownership [a dangerous thing to do, I would have thought] and unnecessarily harassing a patient abut firearm ownership"—for example, by constantly reminding him that it is dangerous to leave a loaded gun lying around within reach of a child.

The law, called the Firearm Owners' Privacy Act, was challenged because it was said to be in breach of the First Amendment's prohibition on the curtailment of free speech. The law seems to me to have been *prima facie* preposterous, an unwarrantable intrusion into the professional conduct of doctors. In fact it was overturned, but on shaky grounds, I thought. It was held that the law would have been warranted if it could have been shown to increase patient safety; but of course it could not.

The authors of the article state that the majority on the court of appeals held that "laws regulating physician speech must be designed to enhance rather than harm patient safety." The authors then go on to cite evidence that gun ownership in the home "increases the risk of death for all household members, especially the risk of death by suicide," and "the majority of U.S. adults who live in homes with guns are unaware of the heightened risk posed by bringing guns into a home." From this the authors conclude that "a physician's counseling can not only enhance a patient's capacity for self-determination, but also save lives."

Then comes the rather sinister bit: "Given the right to provide such counsel, professional norms recognize the responsibility to do so." In the space of a couple of paragraphs, we have gone from proscriptive censorship to prescriptive censorship, from what you *cannot* say to what you *must* say. One wonders how long it will be before a parent whose infant kills himself by shooting himself with a loaded gun left lying about in the home sues his doctor for not having warned him of the danger as he should have done. And on the worldview here expressed, all adults fundamentally remain infants, unless they are in authority.

Prescriptive censorship is much more destructive of free speech than proscriptive, because it is harder to get around by Aesopian language, though it can still be ridiculed, for example by gross and obvious exaggeration. But one cannot help wondering whether the reaction against it would have been so strong of the Florida legislature had chosen other subjects for proscriptive censorship of physicians—if perhaps it had forbidden doctors to tell the lie, peddled by the National Institute on Drug Abuse, that addiction is a chronic relapsing brain condition. The test of a person's commitment to freedom is not if he protests when his own freedom is curtailed, but when that of someone with whom he disagrees is curtailed. ◼

May 25, 2017

The use of substances derived from cannabis for medical purposes (if they are therapeutically useful) has never seemed to me to present any particular ethical problems. There are, of course, practical problems, since cannabis contains more than a hundred substances, each of which needs to be tested separately. But almost certainly, scientific trials will help to demystify a plant that for so long has been the botanical *fer de lance* of counterculture in the West. Substances derived from cannabis will go through the cycle of attitudes to new drugs described in the textbook of pharmacology that I used as a student: first miracle cure, then deadly poison, and finally useful in some cases.

In this week's *Journal* there is a controlled trial of cannabidiol, a purified derivative of the plant, for the treatment of Dravet syndrome, a tragic childhood disorder that consists of serious mental retardation and intractable epilepsy. Reports that cannabis reduces the frequency and severity of epileptic attacks have been numerous but anecdotal; disbelievers disbelieve because they suspect that the anecdotes are but stalking horses for a relaxation or total abandonment of controls on the drug. No one would use cannabidiol for pleasure, however. Here it was used in a double-blind trial in 120 children and adolescents with Dravet syndrome, a condition fortunately so rare that the researchers had to search twenty-three institutions across the world to find the patients.[1]

---

1 Rare conditions are fortunate for drug companies too. Orphan diseases are those so rare that they would not normally attract pharmaceutical companies to research remedies for them. But if they do find such a remedy, the life of the drug's patent is

They observed the numbers of fits from which the patients suffered for a period of four weeks before the start of the trial, and then in the subsequent fourteen weeks when they were given either cannabidiol or placebo. The results were quite clear: cannabidiol did reduce the frequency of fits. In the first month, the median number of fits declined in the treatment group from 12.4 to 5.0, whereas in the placebo group it declined only from 14.9 to 13. This difference was highly significant (statistically, if not necessarily in any other way). By the end of the trial, three of the patients taking cannabidiol were entirely free of fits but none of those taking placebo was.

There was one result, however, that struck me as rather odd. While 43 percent of those taking cannabidiol had the number of their fits reduced by at least 50 percent, 27 percent of those taking placebo likewise had the number of their fits reduced by at least 50 percent. This suggests either a very strong placebo effect, or that the natural fluctuations in the number of fits in this condition are very strong, in which case the result from cannabidiol seems somewhat less impressive. Indeed, the natural variation in the number of fits is immense: among the patients given cannabidiol, it ranged from 3.9 fits per month to 1,717 fits per month before treatment, and afterward from zero fits to 2,159. This means that fits must have increased in frequency from 2.56 per hour to 3.21 per hour under cannabidiol in at least one patient.[2]

There were also more "adverse events" with cannabidiol than with placebo, and thus nine patients under treatment withdrew from the trial whereas only three of those under placebo did so. The odd thing about the nature of adverse events in the trial was that they were of precisely the same kind in both the treatment and the placebo groups. Surely one might have expected some difference between them?

---

extended to compensate the company for the small number of patients who will take it. The trick is subsequently to find that the remedy is of much wider application than first thought. And the patent can be indefinitely extended by finding new orphan diseases that are remedied or ameliorated by the drug. More than one drug company has made a fortune this way. Without this system, no one would bother with Dravet's syndrome, devastating as it is. The study in the *Journal* was designed and financed by the company that manufactures cannabidiol. This, of course, does not imply any dishonesty.

2   The huge variation in the number of fits between the patients must cast some doubt on the value and validity of the analysis and conclusions.

Overall, cannabidiol was of some benefit, but was certainly no panacea. From the point of view of the drug company, at any rate, it was a success, at least until something better comes along. As ever, further research needs to be done.

⸺

When it comes to medically assisted dying, my views are both inconsistent and fluctuating. I approve of it for myself, as I fear being reduced to the condition that I have witnessed in many patients. On the other hand, I cannot help but think that there is something to the thin-end-of-the-wedge or slippery-slope argument. I have seen grasping relatives desperate for the death of their supposedly loved one, the sooner to inherit, and I have seen doctors and hospital managers frustrated at the persistent occupation of hospital beds by those whom they consider would be better off dead. When it comes to those who view themselves in that way, one suspects that there will soon be pressure for an inalienable right to medically assisted dying for anyone who wants it. Is not a good death a fundamental human right, and why should you have to be already ill in order to exercise it? That would be a form of discrimination, which is now believed to be bad even when properly and necessarily employed.

Another paper in the *Journal* this week describes the efforts of the University Health Network in Toronto to implement a "hospital-based program" to provide "medical assistance in dying" after it was made legal in Canada. The acronym used there is MAiD, and I think the word "in" was added to the common term "medically assisted dying" so as to avoid the acronym MAD.

If, as Buffon said, the style is the man himself, then the man who wrote this paper—or rather, the committee, for there are seven authors—was uneasy about it. The language is relentlessly bureaucratic in style, if bureaucratese has a style. Here is a sample: "Institution-based delivery and the hospital-wide education process surrounding it have brought assisted dying more prominently into the public space of medical care." The word *intervention* is repeatedly used for the provision of the means by which a patient can kill himself, and that term has—for me, at any rate—the ring of *Sonderbehandlung*, the special treatment whose specialness turned out to be the gassing of mental patients. And *program* doesn't quite seem the right word for what is being done, either.

In the Toronto hospitals reported on here, 74 patients made inquiries about putting themselves down with medical assistance. Of these, 45 essentially excluded themselves by dying in the meantime, or by changing their minds, or by lacking the capacity to choose to die. That left 29 in the "program." Of these, 19 were permitted, granted or supplied with the "intervention." Why the others were not is unspecified.

I could not help but notice that 18 of those 19 were white and had relatively large incomes. Surely, rich old whites were overrepresented in the sample? There are two possible ways to address this inequity. The first is to deny the rich old whites their privileged access to easeful death; the other is to enroll poor members of underprivileged ethnic minorities in the "program," either by educative means or—if those fail to produce the desired result of ethnic equality among the medically assisted moribund—by conscription. Generations of disadvantage have left those minorities mistrustful. Give affirmative action a chance!

I noticed also that in this MAiD program, only intravenous drugs were used; oral preparations were thought to be less reliable in their outcome. With this, I think, hardly anyone could quarrel. But does it not seem odd that a perfectly painless and certain death is possible by these means in the context of MAiD, but not, apparently, in that of executions in the United States, in the course of which all kinds of horrors have been reported where they have been carried out by injection? I suppose the difference between death by injection in MAiD and that in capital punishment is analogous to the difference between arranged and forced marriage. One is freely entered into and the other is not. ▣

June 1, 2017

Some of the most fatal words—fatal, that is, in their ultimate effect— appeared in the letters column of the *Journal* on January 10, 1980. The five-sentence letter by Porter and Jick led to, or perhaps I should say was followed by, the deaths of at least 183,000 people by overdose of prescription opioids from 1999 to 2015, to which nearly 80,000 can now be added from 2016 and 2017.

The letter was titled "Addiction Rare in Patients Treated with Narcotics," and it pointed out that very few patients treated in hospital with drugs like morphine for severe acute pain became addicted to them. This is certainly true in my experience; and looking at the question from the other end of the telescope, I did not come across a single heroin addict among the hundreds who were my patients (if only briefly) who addicted themselves through having been treated with opiates in hospital for a condition causing acute pain. In Britain, unlike the United States, opioids are rarely given to patients attending emergency departments who do not require admission to hospital.

The correspondence column this week returns to the Porter and Jick letter. It analyzes the fate, as it were, of that letter, which could in retrospect be compared to that of a delayed-action explosive. The authors of the new letter, who are Canadian, counted the citations of Porter and Jick year by year after its publication, and divided them into those that were affirmatory of the original letter, those that were contradictory, and those that were neither. In this context, contradictory means denying that the finding that patients treated in hospital very rarely became addicted to narcotics is a good reason for treating all those who suffer chronic pain with narcotics since (supposedly) they will not become addicted to them.

The number of citations remained low until 1989, when there was a big uptick, and then reached a sustained peak between 1996 and 2002. The overwhelming majority of citations were affirmatory. The first citation contradicting the supposed lesson of the original letter appeared in 1999—that is, nineteen years later—and it was only a single instance. There was another single instance in 2001. In the same years, there were twenty-three and twenty-five affirmatory citations, respectively. It was not until 2017, in fact, that negative citations outnumbered positive ones, and by that time there had been many more than 200,000 deaths from overdoses of prescription opioids. According to the authors, there had not been a single affirmatory citation so far in 2017.

This seems to me extraordinary. Even as late as 2009, when the pattern of deaths had become clear, there were nine affirmatory citations and none in contradiction. I assume, of course, that the authors of the recent letter have been diligent in their searches and truthful in their reporting of their findings. Mistrust has to stop somewhere.

The whole episode is a very curious one—if curious is a word that is not too weak to apply to something associated with (if not actually the sole cause of) so many deaths. The fact is that any reasonably experienced doctor should have known from the outset that the findings on a group of hospital patients with acute pain, such as that caused by heart attack, peritonitis, surgery and so forth, were not to be applied uncritically to the assorted group of patients with chronic backache and other long-lasting grumbling pains of uncertain etiology. I never mistook the one for the other, and I don't consider it to be much of an achievement.

Authors are not to be held responsible for the use to which their words are put, even when they are clearly inflammatory and meant as such. It takes two for inflammatory words to inflame, and while inflammatory words are not admirable, they do not absolve the inflamed from their responsibility for their subsequent actions. In like fashion, expert witnesses are sometimes blamed for miscarriages of justice because they misled the court; but it is precisely to test evidence that courts are established, and if they fail to do so adequately the blame is theirs rather than that of the experts. The expert is to be reprehended only if he is dishonest, and even then is less responsible for any miscarriage of justice than the court that accepted his lies or misrepresentations.

This new letter, no doubt deliberately, raises more questions than it answers, or sets out to answer. Why did so many years elapse before much notice was taken of Porter and Jick? Why was there such overwhelming support for a point of view that was almost self-evidently wrong? And why did it take so many scores of thousands of deaths for the worm finally to turn?

It seems to me likely that notice was taken of Porter and Jick only once strong oral semisynthetic opioid drugs became available in the 1990s. To have suggested before then that patients with chronic pain should routinely be given injections of morphine or heroin would have seemed ludicrous even to the most gullible. But still that does not explain the overwhelming predominance of publications favorably disposed to the prescription of strong opioids to those in chronic pain, with the supposedly reassuring support of (if not necessarily because of) Porter and Jick, and the absence of significant opposition.

There are two main explanations, not mutually exclusive. The first is that there was a commercially inspired campaign that confounded medical literature with advertising. The second is that those in favor of prescribing opioids to people with chronic pain were evangelical about it, while those who were against it had no fervor; they thought it self-evidently wrong and simply refrained from prescribing, without making a fuss about it. So a false aura of consensus was created, all affirmation and no denial.

The fact is that most doctors most of the time are ruled in their practice by professional consensus, of necessity, because they do not have the time to investigate the evidence behind everything that they do, unless they happen to be super-specialized. They are not exactly obeying orders, but they are certainly following fashion, good and bad. Is this right for a learned or liberal profession? It is not ideal, perhaps, but it is probably unavoidable. Knowledge, and certainly information, expands so fast that no renaissance man can keep up with more than an infinitesimal portion of it. A doctor skims the journals and does what they suggest.

Though he cannot possibly hope to justify everything he does if called upon to do so, the doctor is still held responsible for everything he does. Indeed, if anything he grows ever more responsible for what he does. In English law, it used to be a doctor's defense against an accusation of negligence that a body of responsible doctors would have acted in the circumstances exactly as he acted, but this is no longer sufficient. What the body of responsible doctors would do has itself to be reasonable, *sub specie aeternitatis* as it were. The doctor can no longer rely on the argument from authority: he cannot point to this letter of June 2017, for example, and say that the vast majority of what was published in the medical literature was in support of what he did, because the vast majority of what was published in the medical literature on this subject was rubbish. And not only was it rubbish, it was *obviously* rubbish.

That it took so long to expose it as such is perhaps harder to explain. The fact that a large body of educated and intelligent people can have allowed the situation to continue for so long should be enough to caution anyone from merely accepting a consensus among such people as being necessarily much more enlightened than the vaporings of barroom philosophers. Perhaps it continued for so long because the problem, though a large and important one, was highly concentrated, and concentrated precisely in those areas in which doctors had the most to lose by exposing it. The better doctors, having no experience of it as a problem, had no pressing reason to expose it when it was not happening on their back doorstep.

Is there any defense against such a thing happening again? The only defense that I can see is: a) an intelligently critical attitude to what one reads, and b) publications that do not readily surrender to consensus. By an intelligently critical attitude, I do not mean the rejection of all consensus *because* it is consensus. Fortunately, not all consensus is wrong. The trick, the art, the science, is knowing when it is and why. ◾

June 8, 2017

In general, rich people are healthier than poor people. This is not an invariable rule—invariable rules are hard to come by in medicine—and rich people may die young. If official statistics are to be believed, Cubans die old but they do not live rich; and when I used to visit the tiny Pacific island of Nauru, it was one of the richest countries in the world (thanks to its phosphate resources) but its citizens certainly did not have a long life expectancy. All the same, as generalizations go, this is a good one.

An article in this week's *Journal* draws attention to an epidemiological paradox in the United States: while the incidence among whites of four cancers, those of the breast, prostate, thyroid and skin (melanoma), are 50 percent higher in rich areas than in poor, death rates are more or less identical and declining. A graph shows that the incidence began greatly to diverge from about 1990.

What explains this paradox? As ever, there is more than one possible explanation. Suppose for a moment that the difference in incidence were real: that it actually reflected what was occurring within the respective populations. It could be that the superior medical treatment received by the rich canceled out the difference in incidence, to result in the same death rate. But this is not the explanation favored by the authors, nor does it seem very likely.

The four selected cancers have indolent forms, which are very slow-growing. It is often said (truly) that more men die *with* cancer of the prostate than *of* it: a very high percentage of men dying above the age of

eighty of other causes also have cancer of the prostate as what patholo-
gists call an incidental finding. Therefore, if doctors examine rich
patients more often and more closely than they examine the poor, they
are likely to find more indolent cancers (which would probably not end
up killing the patient). This is to the disadvantage of the rich, because
the finding of such harmless cancers is not without consequences: the
patient becomes anxious, and is subjected to tests and operations that
do no good but can do harm. They are also a waste of money.

I noticed that the words *injustice* and *inequity* are nowhere used in
this connection, as they would almost certainly have been if the figures
had shown that the incidence of the four cancers was higher among the
poor. This suggests a belief that no injustice can be done to the rich, or
that justice is not due them because they are rich—an attitude that in
the twentieth century was as baleful as were similar attitudes to people
of a different race.

Screening programs, no doubt intensifying in the 1990s, are probably a cause of the disparity to the disadvantage of the rich in America.
The authors propose that "systems serving relatively wealthy and
healthy populations may see offering more testing as a good way to
attract consumers, produce more patients, and increase business." I
think it would be vain to deny that this might well be true. If you offer
a doctor a fee to perform a service, it is more likely that he will perform
that service. But this is far from the whole truth.

In their opening sentence, the authors refer in the following words
to a famous British study of health and wealth:

> Income has long been known to be an important determinant of
> health. Four decades ago, the Whitehall study of British civil servants
> revealed that higher employment grades were associated with better
> physical and mental health and lower mortality.

If you read this passage carefully, and do not just slide your mind over it
as perhaps you are intended to do, you will note that the authors beat a
retreat in the second sentence from the claim made in the first, a retreat
necessary in the interests of strict accuracy. In the first sentence income
is held to be a *determinant* of health, but in the second it is held only to
be *associated* with health; because, of course, the higher grades in the

civil service differ from the lower by more than just their income (or so one would hope). They differ in intelligence, levels of education, heredity, daily habits and no doubt in many other things, such as the degree to which they took warnings against smoking to heart and conformed their conduct to their knowledge. But in the matter of access to health care, at least in theory, they were no better off, no more privileged than the poor, thanks to Britain's socialized medical system.[1]

I suspect that the same pattern of differential incidence of the four cancers would be found in Britain as in the United States: that it was higher among the richer than the poorer parts of the population, though the death rates were similar. And this would be so despite the fact that the system of incentives for doctors in Britain is different from that in America.

The difference is in the behavior of patients. Richer patients are usually better educated than poor patients. They are more concerned with their health and more likely to seek and comply with medical advice. In the instance of screening for these four cancers, this works, unusually, to their disadvantage. (The authors of the article, incidentally, do not state whether their statistics are age-adjusted, an important epidemiological consideration that might profoundly alter them.)

I am glad to report that the authors end their article with words of wisdom that are rare these days:

> Although we [the medical profession] have much to offer people who are sick or injured, physicians have overstated medicine's role in promoting health. In so doing, we may have unintentionally devalued the role of more important determinants of health for people of every income level—healthy food, regular movement, and finding purpose in life.

In short, what the early eighteenth-century physicians, such as George Cheyne, called *regimen*. It is curious how, in the welter of change, some things remain the same.

---

1 This is not absolutely true because, unlike in Canada, private medical care is not prohibited. It probably accounts for no more than 5 or 10 percent of all medical care, and a much smaller proportion than this in the case of screening for the four cancers mentioned in this article.

〜

I offer no prizes for those who guess the tenor of the article titled "Health Effects of the Recent Presidential Election." The title is somewhat misleading, however, because the article does not confine itself to the health effects of the election per se, but also delves into the supposed effects of racial or cultural prejudice in general.

Oddly enough, the authors quote evidence from the aftermath of the events at Duke University in which a black female student falsely accused some white male students of rape and racial denigration of her. Thereafter, apparently, black female students at the university showed heightened biochemical responses to stress. But whose fault, one might ask, was that? The alleged racism of the falsely accused, or the false witness of the black student who made the allegation? Personally, I have no difficulty whatever in believing that it is stressful and harmful to health and well-being to be the object of prejudice and hatred; but if this is the case, those who seek to exaggerate or even fabricate episodes of such prejudice and hatred, and give them publicity knowing them to be false, are themselves responsible for causing the same affects.

There are other peculiarities in the article. It points out that illegal immigrants feel stressed when they fear deportation, and they experience physiological changes caused by that stress. I do not doubt that this is true. But I am certain that the same might be said of burglars or murderers when they have cause to believe that the police are on their track. Are we to say that the police should therefore desist from trying to capture them? Does personal distress trump all other considerations?

One may wonder, if Mrs. Clinton had won the election instead of Mr. Trump, whether we would have seen a similar article measuring the cortisol levels of those she consigned to her basket of deplorables. ◼

June 15, 2017

A paper in this week's *Journal* begins rather discouragingly: "Health care in the United States is extremely costly. There is compelling evidence that a large share of spending—particularly in Medicare—results in little or no patient benefit."

If a considerable amount of medical activity has no benefit, it is not, of course, unique in its uselessness: it has long been my belief that a very high proportion of the human activity known as work is useless or worse. This was illustrated in the 1970s when the working week in Britain was reduced from five days to three because of a miners' strike that reduced coal supplies to coal-fired electricity generators. Total economic output declined not by a proportionate 40 percent, but only by 20 percent, thus proving that at least one day a week at work under normal circumstances was devoted to doing nothing, or nothing productive. Presence at work is not the same as production. Americans in particular are prone to the superstition that working eighty hours a week results in twice as much productive activity as working forty and that longer holidays are necessarily bad for productivity. But output does not grow proportionately with input either of time or of money, and hence arises the wasteful medical spending lamented in the paper with the dismal beginning (to which I will return shortly). I assume, of course, that the ostensible aim of health care is its principle aim, which may in fact not be the case.

One of the reasons advanced for the high cost and inefficiency of the American health-care system is its comparatively undeveloped primary care. This explanation is put forward in an essay titled "A Tale of Two Doctors—Structural Inequalities and the Culture of Medicine." The author, herself a doctor, relates her different experience of consulting a family doctor and an orthopedic surgeon. She points out that the median annual incomes of the two types of doctors are $193,776 and $525,000 respectively, so it is hardly surprising that debt-laden medical students would opt for the higher-paid specialty as a career, irrespective of whether they have a vocation for it. The better-paid specialists, moreover, have an instinctual or at least second-nature inclination to prefer expensive and technologically sophisticated approaches to problems that might have easier solutions.

I used to be somewhat skeptical of the value of primary care or family doctors. When I have something wrong with my leg, why should I not go straight to the orthopedic surgeon rather than passing through primary care first? Does this not waste my time and lead to frustration and even to avoidable suffering?

Since meeting several American friends who have no family doctors and no money problems, I have changed my mind. In their cases, the absence of a coordinating family doctor resulted in polypharmacy, repetition of unnecessary investigations, neglect of the most obvious considerations, redundant consultations, and a strange and elaborate form of negligence involving an excess of concern and a dearth of reflection. Just as those who protect their children from the most risks are not necessarily the best parents, so medical care is not best because of its sheer volume.

Near the end of her article, the author imagines a Martian landing in the United States and contemplating what our present health-care system says about us. The visitor, she writes, might

> conclude that we prefer treatment to prevention, that our skin and bones matter more to us than our children or sanity, that patient benefit is not a prerequisite for approved use of treatments or procedures, that drugs always work better than exercise, that doctors treat computers not people, that death is avoidable with the right care, that hospitals are the best place to be sick, and that we value avoiding wrinkles or warts more than we do hearing, chewing, or walking.

There is much to discuss, to agree or disagree with, in this sentence, with all its connotations, implications and imputations. For example, it is by no means always absurd to prefer treatment to prevention, if prevention comes at too high a price, as it often does. To complain that people are concerned about their appearance rather than about deeper realities is to complain of human nature, and almost to lament that humans are social beings. There is the implication that sanity is procurable by medical means, just because *in*sanity is medically treatable; personally, I believe that the very notion of *mental health* is productive of untold and avoidable misery. But overall, the sentence is an eloquent plea for a more humane practice of medicine—and which of us has not encountered a doctor seemingly more interested in his computer screen than in the patient who consults him?

As for improving the cost-effectiveness of health care, another approach is described in the *NEJM* paper I quoted at the beginning of this section, titled "Changes in Hospital Quality Associated with Hospital Value-Based Purchasing." The authors attempted to assess the effect of Hospital Value-Based Purchasing (HVBP), whereby hospitals would be paid for treating Medicare patients for certain acute diseases if their overall outcomes met a previously laid-down standard of success. Would the standard of care in hospitals paid in this way improve more than in hospitals not paid in this way?

The diseases selected for payment in this fashion were heart attack, heart failure and pneumonia. The authors compared the improvement in outcomes in those hospitals paid by HVBP and those not paid by it. There was no statistically significant difference in the results for the first two diseases, and only a small difference for the third. Moreover, the results did not permit the conclusion that outcomes were superior for hospitals paid by HVBP *because* they were paid by HVBP. In short, the results do not provide evidence that HVBP improves outcomes.

Personally, I did not find these results in the least surprising. It was to hospitals as organizations, not to doctors and nurses as individuals, that the incentive applied. Moreover, it was a negative rather than a positive incentive, a stick rather than a carrot.

Having said that "HVBP...has resulted in little tangible benefit over its first 4 years," the authors go on to say: "It is possible that alternative incentive designs—including those with simpler criteria for performance and larger financial incentives—might have led to greater improvement among hospitals." But in fact there are strong objections to all attempts to raise general standards of care by such means.

In the first place, there is an element of chance in results of treatment in hospitals; those results do not simply reflect the skill and devotion of medical staff, and nothing else. When neonatal units in Britain were ranked by result, it was found that the ranking varied year by year in a random fashion: units would appear to be good in one year and bad the next, and vice versa. The task of setting appropriate standards, so that hospitals are not unfairly penalized by the operations of chance, is neither an easy nor a straightforward one.

Second, only *certain* of a hospital's activities are targeted and measured in this way. If there is a strong enough incentive for hospitals to reach targets for *those* activities, the entire effort of the hospital might be distorted to the detriment of the other activities. If, on the other hand, *all* the hospital's activities were targeted and measured in this way, a bureaucratic monster would have to be created, dwarfing all previous bureaucratic monsters. It never seems to be fully appreciated that measurement itself has a cost, often a very considerable one. Trying to prove one's efficiency can get in the way of one's efficiency.

Third, where there is government payment by results, results are often achieved by bureaucratic manipulation rather than in reality. The consequence is a generalized intellectual and moral corruption.

Fourth, if the targets laid down are too stringent, so that some hospitals (not necessarily through any fault of their own) are unable to meet them, they may actually depress standards rather than raise them. If you will be punished for not meeting standards that you know that you cannot meet, why even try?

As a means of raising standards of medical care in general, then, payment by results is open to *prima facie* objections. In my view, general standards rise more because of technical advance than because of anything even remotely like HVBP. Treatment of peptic ulceration has improved all over the world beyond all recognition not because of any incentives, positive or negative, given to doctors or hospitals, but because the previously unknown cause was discovered by two Australian researchers. The cause was easily treated and the treatment spread around the world in very short order; it was self-evidently beneficial. Very few people now suffer from peptic ulceration in the way that was commonplace well within living memory. No incentive, other than most doctors' desire to do the best for their patients, was necessary to raise the standard of care in this disease. ◙

June 22, 2017

As a former prison doctor myself, I was particularly interested this week in an article titled "On Incarceration and Health—Reframing the Discussion." I knew more or less what to expect and I was not disappointed: a mixture of high-flown sentiment, truisms (which are truisms, nevertheless, because they are true) and statements that are, to say the least, disputable.

The article is built around the case of Mr. P., a man who "had spent more than half of his life" in a maximum-security prison, San Quentin in California. Mr. P. had cancer of some kind that required chemotherapy; he had recently shouted "profanities" at a prison nurse, who reported him to the authorities, who in response lengthened his sentence by three months.

The article does not favor us with an account of Mr. P.'s criminal record, and the reader's emotional dice are loaded by this omission. He could be imprisoned for anything from being the victim of a miscarriage of justice to the serial sexual killing of children. If Mr. P. is guilty of the latter, most readers would be relieved to know that he eventually spent more than half his life in prison, and few would doubt that he deserved it.

Still, the general point of the author, that prisoners should as far as possible be treated with dignity, and should be given proper health care, is one with which I agree. There are those who want to make prison a prolonged Calvary, presumably on the grounds that this would render it more of a deterrent both to the prisoners when (or if) released and to the rest of society. But efficacy in itself—assuming for a moment that such a policy is empirically effective—is not a complete justification of any given punishment. To cut off the arms and legs of shoplifters would surely be efficacious, but it would be barbaric, and barbarism is to be avoided simply because it is barbarism.

Certainly, the cell in which Mr. P. was held sounds cruelly spartan, especially if he is to continue living there for an extended time. "There was no mirror in his cell," writes the author, though it is just possible that there was no mirror because he had in the past broken mirrors and used the shards either as a weapon or to harm himself. Prison authorities are often criticized for failing to prevent suicides or injuries to others by not keeping the means away from the prisoners.

The nurse at whom he had shouted profanities was shocked by the harshness of the penalty inflicted on him for having done so. "Even with her limited experience working in prison, she understood that lengthening Mr. P.'s incarceration was harmful to his health."

Irrespective of whether the additional sentence was either just or justified in this particular case, the writer evidently thinks that the first concern of the criminal justice system is, or ought to be, the convicted lawbreaker's health. If punishment is bad for his health, then it ought not to be inflicted. As it happens, the next paragraph calls for more attention to the health consequences of incarceration itself:

> With the rise in mass incarceration, the biomedical community has become increasingly interested in investigating such determinants of incarceration as addiction and mental health disorders. Less attention has been paid to the ways in which incarceration itself is harmful to health. This neglect is at least partly attributable to the fact that official statistics don't accurately capture the lived experience of inmates. For example, statistics show that mortality among people living in prisons and jails is lower than that among the general adult population.

Now, mortality is not the only possible measure of health, but it is an important one, and at least a fairly reliable one, death being so objectively measurable an outcome. In other circumstances, it would be unusual to argue that lower mortality did not indicate better health. The sound of special pleading is here clearly audible.

A little later in the article, the author cites the study of British civil servants—the same one cited in the *Journal* two weeks earlier—showing that the higher grades, who had more scope for independent action and control over their work, lived longer than the lower grades, who merely followed orders, even when such factors as blood pressure, obesity and diabetes were taken into account. "These studies," says our author, "were the first to definitively show that people in lower social classes had higher rates of premature death than those in higher classes, despite equal access to health care." And the supposed reason for the disparity "lies in autonomy and social participation," which almost by definition is very low in prisons everywhere, prisoners being subject to the authority of their guards even in very small matters. From the point of view of personal autonomy and control over one's own life, being a prisoner is worse, even, than being a lower-echelon British civil servant.

While I can easily imagine that a low level of personal autonomy leads to frustration and thereby to relatively poor health, I can also easily imagine the near-opposite: that for some people, at least, the demand or necessity that they should take control of their own lives is threatening and anxiety-provoking, and therefore bad for health. That explains, perhaps, why some prisoners, at least in Britain, preferred life in prison to life outside; they felt safer inside, not only from others but from themselves. We are not all cut from the same cloth, and it is an elementary mistake to suppose that what we consider good for ourselves must be good for everyone else.

As we have seen earlier, the statistics on mortality for prisoners in Britain, by comparison with the social class in which prisoners are mostly born, show that they would be nearly twice as likely to die if they were left at liberty. This is so even though in theory they have "equal access to health care" outside prison, and even though the suicide rate in prison is several times that of the nonincarcerated. At first sight it may be surprising that prison should be a kind of health resort of the slums, but it accords with my experience. The article itself halfway suggests the reasons, saying that "a lower risk of death may indicate that incarceration often forcibly removes people from dangerous cir-cumstances." This is a revealing way of putting it. For the author, the prisoners have circumstances, but do not actively participate in them, let alone create them.

What are the dangerous circumstances from which prisoners are forcibly removed by their incarceration? An important one must be the taking of drugs. In the fifteen years in which I served as a doctor in prison, not a single prisoner died of an overdose of drugs, which certainly would not have been the case with a similar group of people outside prison. If you regard taking drugs as merely an illness rather than the expression of human volition and decision, imprisonment "removes people from dangerous circumstances" as if from a contaminated water supply. But apart from being empirically mistaken, does this not deny them the very agency the lack of which is supposed to be so harmful to them as prisoners? The reason that prisoners have a lower mortality rate in prison than they would have at liberty is that they *do* things that are deleterious to their health when they are free to do them.

Of course, human choices are influenced by "circumstances," chief among them being the culture in which those humans live. But this, almost certainly, is not what the author had in mind, for he would almost certainly subscribe to the pieties of multiculturalism according to which no way of life is better than any other.

That prisoners should actually be healthier inside prison than out, even when health care is available to them at no cost to themselves, is hardly a comforting thought. For many of them, prison is the *only* place in which they receive proper health care, because of their choices, priorities and conduct outside prison. They need Socrates, not evasive, exculpatory claptrap. ◾

June 29, 2017

When I was a young boy in London, we had fogs in November so thick—they were known as pea-soupers—that we could not see our hands when we held them up before our eyes. Men had to walk in front of vehicles to guide them on their way. I still remember the buses, all lights on, looming up out of the fog from only a few yards away, with a man walking before them like a mourner before a hearse.

I loved those fogs and looked forward to them eagerly. They seemed to me so exciting, and I missed them when the Clean Air Act consigned them rapidly to the past. I did not know that they probably killed several thousand people, and I am not absolutely sure that my childish regret at their passing would have been any the less *had* I known it. A child is a natural egotist.

No adult would want his air polluted, even if polluted air had no adverse health consequences, because air pollution is aesthetically unpleasant. Air pollution has declined in the most advanced nations in the world, thanks to regulation of emissions and more efficient energy generation and manufacturing processes; though perhaps some of the improvement has been caused by the export of manufacturing to the workshops of the world, particularly China. Our ability to import cheap goods from China (and elsewhere) must depend to an extent on the ability of manufacturers there to ignore the costs imposed by environmental protection. Anyone who has been to a large Chinese or Indian city will understand that air pollution is now so serious a problem that it is beginning to erode economic efficiency.

The inhabitants of those cities now breathe contaminated air so that we may live cheaply.

The quality of our air having improved, is its level of pollution now so low as to be perfectly safe, with no health effects at all? A long *NEJM* paper sets out to answer the question. In essence, what the authors (from the T. H. Chan School of Public Health at Harvard) did was to correlate the death rates of people with the air pollution levels—small particulate matter and ozone—of the areas in which they lived, defined by ZIP Code. One cannot but admire the authors' industry and diligence, and marvel at the sheer size of their calculations. They worked out the death rates from all causes for all beneficiaries of Medicare in the continental United States from 2000 through 2012, a total of 60,925,443 persons, who on average were receiving Medicare for somewhat more than seven years during that interval. Annual pollution levels were estimated for no fewer than 39,716 ZIP Codes.

In summary, the authors found, or asserted, that each increase in particulate matter of 10 micrograms[1] per cubic meter of air was associated with a 7.3 percent increase in death rate from all causes, and each increase of 10 parts per billion of ozone per cubic meter of air was associated with a 1.1 percent increase in death rate from all causes. The size of the association between concentration of particulate matter and death rate was three times higher for those eligible for Medicaid (a proxy for low socioeconomic status) than it was for the rest of the Medicare population.

What does this mean? The authors had no doubt that it indicates the need for a change in public policy:

> These findings suggest that lowering the National Ambient Air Quality Standards [the permitted levels of pollution] may produce important public health benefits overall, especially among self-identified racial minorities and people with low income.

An editorial accompanying the article is titled "Air Pollution Still Kills," and ends with the rhetorical question *Do we really want to breathe*

---

1 A microgram is a millionth of a gram, and a gram is one 28th of an ounce. Ten micrograms is therefore one 2,800,000th of an ounce.

air that kills us? It is probably fair to say that the correlation found after immense statistical calculations will be widely taken by the readership to be a causative one: the death rate rising with increased air pollution *because* of the air pollution. But correlations in medical research that are founded on observation rather than on experimental manipulation of the variables involved should not be regarded as showing causation except under certain conditions. Only one of those conditions is fulfilled here, namely, consistency with other, similar findings, since no studies have ever found that air pollution is *good* for health.

Another important condition for showing causation is biological plausibility, and here the paper fails. The statistics suggest that the effect of increases in pollution is greater at *lower* levels of pollution than at higher levels, which may be possible but is unlikely. The effects of drugs can indeed be relatively greater at lower levels, so that doubling the effect might require ten times the dose (up to a point). But most of the effects of cigarette smoke are not like that: the total amount of such smoke that you breathe in is linearly related to your chances of getting lung cancer. Other sorts of particulate matter entering the lungs are likely to be comparable in this regard.

The statistical correlation, assuming it arises causatively, showed the effect of air pollution on mortality among people who self-designate as black to be four times greater than for other groups, but is the reason likely to be purely biological?[2] It is possible, but not likely. The authors attempted to control for factors such as obesity, diabetes, and smoking, by analyzing a subset of people for whom these data were available and found that they had no effect on the correlation between death rate and air pollution. This, however, weakens rather than strengthens the chance of a purely biological cause of the increased risk among blacks. If common factors of known, strong biological consequence have no effect on the correlation, then something else—for example crime and violence—must explain it. In any case, exposure to air pollution is far from the main difference, let alone the only difference, between the black population and other parts of the general population.

---

2 I overlook the problems with self-designation. Mr. Obama would undoubtedly have self-designated as black for the purposes of a study such as this, though biologically speaking he is as much white as black. It seems probable, however, that self-designation correlates pretty strongly, though far from perfectly, with race.

The paper has other odd features that should make us extremely wary of its conclusions about a causative relationship. For one, the subjects were (like me) elderly, and 22 million out of the 60-plus million died in the period of study. What the study does not tell us, and what is important to know, is whether the increased risk of death (assuming for the moment that air pollution was entirely causative of the additional deaths) occurred some weeks or some years before they would have died anyway if they had lived in a less polluted area. Was death brought forward by a little or a lot? This is worth knowing, because a single death brought forward by sixty years to the age of twenty is more important (I would say) than a million deaths brought forward by a minute at the age of ninety-five.

There is more. The statement that each increase in particulate matter of 10 micrograms per cubic meter of air was associated with a 7.3 percent increase in death rate from all causes is obviously speculative and open to question, to put it mildly. This is because the concentration of particulate matter in the air across the continental United States varied only from 6.21 to 15.64 micrograms per cubic meter in the first place. The figure of 7.3 percent for the increase in death rate with a 10 microgram per cubic meter increase in particulate matter is therefore an extrapolation, and hence is misleading.

If one analyzed the murder rate in proportion to air pollution, one might find a stronger association. (I am not saying that it *is* so, only that it might be so.) One would not conclude from this that murder was caused by air pollution.

Despite the rather obvious deficiencies of the paper, the editorial says with superb confidence: "The findings...stress the need for tighter regulation of air-pollutant levels, including the imposition of stricter limits on levels of [particulate matter]." The authors of the editorial are fortunate enough to live in a costless world, in which large-scale changes can be imposed without cost and produce only the intended results. Assuming that particulate matter is wholly the product of human endeavor, the authors might with equal justice demand the end of all industrial activity, because there is (according to the paper) *no* safe level of particulate matter in the air. We must return to nature—though, if I have understood correctly, nature does not always deal with us kindly. The state of nature is not one of longevity. ◼

July 6, 2017

When I was very young, we had a single fat boy in the school. His cheeks were so padded that they reduced his eyes to slits; his midriff was so bulky that it necessitated a waddle; his arms and hands stuck out like paddles in the air as he made his slow breathless progress across the playground. It was said to be his glands that accounted for his size; and because he was so unusual, he was plausibly thought to be ill rather than weak-willed or badly brought up. Nowadays he would hardly be thought worthy of notice, so common has such obesity become.

Just over twenty years later, in 1980, I met Professor Paul Zimmett on the Pacific island of Nauru. He was an Australian researcher studying the very high incidence of gross obesity and Type 2 diabetes in the island's population. (The only other group that rivaled them in this respect were the Pima Indians of Arizona.) In the callowness of my youth and inexperience, I thought that he was engaged upon a typical exercise in the academically arcane. I was quite wrong: he was researching the future, not only of these two small and isolated groups but of the whole of humanity.

A long *NEJM* paper titled "Health Effects of Overweight and Obesity in 195 Countries over 25 Years" examines the inexorable rise in obesity worldwide in the years since I met Professor Zimmett. In some countries, my own included, it has been so great that epidemiologists and demographers have suggested that it will halt or even reverse the increase in life expectancy that we have come to accept as the norm. If they are right, our children, and especially our grandchildren, may live shorter lives than ours; but this paper provides some evidence that such pessimism is unwarranted, without going so far as to be positively optimistic.

The authors of the article—all 154 of them, according to my possibly inaccurate count—attempt not only to assess the increase in obesity worldwide between 1980 and 2015, but to estimate its consequences in terms of life expectancy and the number of years that people live with disabilities.

One of the difficulties of such large-scale enterprises is the variability of the quality of the statistics of different countries. Some countries are what Freud would have called anally retentive about their statistics, others cavalier about them or too poor to keep them. The authors try to overcome the difficulties by means of statistical adjustments that the great majority of readers (such as I) will not understand, and whose validity and trustworthiness they will have to take on trust. Faith is an unavoidable necessity in human existence, even in a rational age.

Still, in some respects the figures are clear and speak for themselves. They accord with the experience of common observation. The prevalence of obesity, defined as a body mass index (BMI) of more than 30,[1] has more than doubled since 1980, so that 5 percent of children and 12 percent of adults are obese. The increase among children has been greatest in middle-income countries, "such as China, Brazil and Indonesia."[2] That China and Indonesia should now be regarded as middle-income countries is itself of world-historical interest, for in 1980 they would not have been so considered. Since between them they are home to a quarter of the world's population, this suggests, contrary to the gloomy prognostications prevalent in my youth (and beyond), that the world has become, *grosso modo*, more equal rather than less. Equality in obesity might not be what egalitarians had in mind, but it is nevertheless one sign of equality in a better sense, at least in present circumstances.

---

1 Body mass index (BMI) is the weight of a person in kilograms divided by his height in kilograms squared.

2 I quote the accompanying editorial, titled "Global Health Effect of Overweight and Obesity." In my youth, incidentally, overweight was an adjective only, and not a noun as well.

Obesity tends worldwide to be associated with a high *sociodemographic index*, a composite of a population's income per capita, average educational attainment over the age of fifteen,[3] and total fertility rate. And yet there are obvious exceptions to this rule, if that is what the correlation is taken to be. For example, the highest proportion of obese adults in the world, on a nation-by-nation basis, is in Egypt, where 35.3 percent are obese. Perhaps this has something to do with the policy of subsidizing the price of bread in that country: when I was last there, admittedly a long time ago, it was cheaper to feed chickens bread than the ingredients from which bread was made.

Exceptions make generalizations difficult or inaccurate, such as that wealth increases obesity. It seems to be true that as countries become richer, their populations become fatter, though not in every case. Within countries that are already rich, on the other hand, obesity is associated with poverty, not wealth, though not in every person. In very poor countries—and hence in most of human history—the fat are rich. The poor cannot eat enough to get fat.

The evidence suggests that where obesity is concerned, cure is better than prevention, contrary to the old saw that says the opposite. At least this is the case at present, since *efforts* at prevention have so far failed. If preventive measures were found that proved to be effective, then prevention *would* be better than cure. A problem that one constantly meets in medicine, as elsewhere in human endeavor, is that the wish is often mistaken for the deed or fact. For example, screening procedures are often taken, both by doctors and by patients, to be preventive, because that is what screening procedures are intended to be. Closer examination often demonstrates that screening is a hero with feet of clay, as it were. Similarly, various attempts at preventing obesity have not had the hoped-for result, as the authors acknowledge:

> During the past decade, researchers have proposed a range of interventions to reduce obesity. Among such interventions are restricting the advertisement of unhealthy food to children, improving school

---

3 I suspect that what is measured is years spent in education rather than attainment properly so-called. No doubt there is a correlation between the two, but in rich countries it may be lessening.

meals, using taxation to reduce consumption of unhealthy foods and providing subsidies to increase intake of healthy foods. However, the effectiveness, feasibility of widespread implementation, and sustainability of such interventions need to be evaluated in various settings. In recent years, some countries have started to implement some of these policies, but no major population success has yet been shown.

This does not mean that no policy could ever have such a success, only that so far it has not been found. As the article also says, there is reason to think that obesity in the United States and some other countries has either plateaued or even declined in prevalence in recent years, which suggests that some beneficial cause has probably operated[1]—even if it is only that the population has bethought itself. If this is so, however, it must have bethought itself for a reason: perhaps the publicity given to the epidemic of obesity.

The authors found (after much statistical effort) that the fatal and other consequences of obesity, such as heart attacks, strokes, hypertension and diabetes, have declined since 1980, a decline which partly offsets the harmful consequences of obesity. They attribute this decline to improved medical treatment of the secondary effects of obesity, mostly by means of medication. As for gross obesity itself, the best treatment, or perhaps I should say correction, found so far is surgery.

I was initially puzzled by the following statement in the abstract to the paper: "High BMI accounted for 4.0 million deaths globally, nearly 40% of which occurred in persons who were not obese." I had a vision of fat people killing thin people, perhaps by falling on them from windows or accidentally suffocating them in crowded buses. Then I realized that it meant that people with BMIs between 25 and 30, not obese by medical definition, also died of the consequences of being overweight. ■

---

4 Probably, not certainly. And a projection is not a prediction: just because something has increased or decreased by the same proportion for the last few years does not mean that it will continue to increase until it reaches a saturation point of 100 percent or decline until it reaches zero.

July 13, 2017

"The March of Science—The True Story" is an article defending science as an enterprise. Many thousands of people had marched on Washington in April to defend science against the threat to it supposedly posed by President Trump, which endows him with a greater degree of power than even he, not a person to underestimate his own importance, probably knew that he had.

I am rather doubtful whether science needs defending, least of all from those who attack it. I also doubt whether many would wish to deprive themselves of the obvious benefits of science or question its ability to solve particular problems. Scientism, on the other hand, which is the view that all human questions and problems can be solved by scientific means alone, rightly arouses opposition. Questions of value will, for metaphysical reasons, remain perpetually unsusceptible to scientific answer.

Where science does address questions that are scientifically answerable, its findings are open to challenge and often susceptible to revision, but it does not follow that all scientific consensus is suspect or that the whole enterprise is unreliable. In answering empirical questions it is the most reliable method we have. The author of the article says,

> the justification most people invoke for dismissing scientific consensus that contradicts their beliefs is that science is corrupted—by political meddling, scientists' ambitions, and industry funding.... We hear about experiments that can't be replicated, negative findings that

remain unpublished, and the ubiquity of bias. . . . Academia is lambasted
for an incentive structure favoring quantity over quality, secrecy over
transparency, and exaggeration of the significance of our results.

This all reminds me of the problem of Marxist epistemology, which
holds that people believe what it is in their material interest to believe
rather than what is suggested by objective evidence. As a sociopsychological observation this may often be true, but it is epistemologically
uninteresting. If it is true in the epistemologically interesting sense—
that is to say, *inevitably* and *unavoidably* true—then it is impossible to
know by what standard of truth, other than self-interest, it can be
known to be true. Certainly it did not appear to be in the material self-
interest of those who first put forward the idea.

If all science is corrupted by self-interest or ideological bias, by
what standard of truth could it be demonstrated, since the supposed
corruption by self-interest or ideological bias must apply to that very
observation? No scientific evidence could be adduced to show that all
science is tainted, for that evidence would itself be tainted—just as the
existence of optical illusion cannot establish that all visual experience
is illusory, for the illusion itself would then be illusory.

The author writes that "remarkable gains in human longevity are
just one manifestation of science's success," an assertion which is certainly open to historical criticism. Scientific progress has in the past
been neither a necessary nor a sufficient condition for the elimination
of disease, for example. According to Thomas McKeown, a famous
epidemiologist, death rates in Western Europe and North America,
and deaths from epidemic diseases, started to decline well before there
was any scientific treatment for them[1] and even before their causes

---

1 A prime example of this was tuberculosis. By the time the first drug known to be
   effective against it, streptomycin, was developed, the death rate from tuberculosis had
   already fallen by something like 95 percent from its peak. Of course, there had been
   many other attempted treatments, such as surgically induced pneumothorax, which
   are generally disparaged from the modern standpoint. But their effectiveness can
   now never be known, because no one would conduct a properly controlled trial of
   them, and such trials were never performed in their own day. It might be that some
   of the remedies—including arsenical compounds—really *were* effective, or partially
   effective. Absence of proof of efficacy is not proof of absence of efficacy. But the
   generally accepted explanation of the decline in mortality from tuberculosis is an
   improvement in nutrition and living conditions. I leave it to economic historians to
   decide how far scientific advance accounts for that improvement.

were known. Nevertheless, the startling transformation, well within living memory, in the fate of millions who once would have suffered for years or even whole lifetimes from peptic ulceration is due entirely to science. Recently, having had an attack of gout, I was relieved of the pain with greater speed and efficacy than anyone who had had such an attack at the time of my birth would have been; moreover, I can now prevent future attacks almost entirely by taking every day a pill that is more or less free of side effects. This is entirely on account of scientific advance.

The author's conclusion is largely but not entirely right, and is a little more tentative than necessary, at least where medicine is concerned. Karl Popper, the philosopher of science, stressed that what distinguishes science from non-science is the falsifiability of its hypotheses, and that no evidence in favor of such hypotheses can ever establish their truth once and for all, only their non-falsity so far. Therefore, scientific doctors have nothing to be ashamed of when they change their opinion about something, even if it is a diametrical change. Indeed, this is a strength, not a weakness: they are following the evidence rather than dogma.

The author says that scientists must "learn to tell stories that emphasize that what makes science right is the enduring capacity to admit we are wrong." In general, I concur; but I also think that this slightly overstates the degree to which the findings of science are provisional—an impression that is bound to be increased by reading the medical journals that specialize, after all, in exploring the frontiers of the unknown. Some findings are indeed refuted by new findings, and the prevailing view on some questions will change; no one will have failed to notice that scientific dietary advice alters regularly and sometimes seems to go round in circles. But no one seriously expects any researcher now to find that the blood does *not* circulate in the body, or that insulin is *not* produced in the pancreas. Some things are known for good and all.

Another problem facing doctors is that patients like certainty. On the few occasions when I have been seriously ill and nigh unto death, I wanted my doctor to know exactly what to do, and to know it on a rational basis. Patientkind cannot bear very much uncertainty. Unfortunately, life and science are often not as unequivocal as we should like. Two papers in this week's *Journal* illustrate this truth.

The first concerns adjuvant therapy in certain cases of cancer of the breast. In this trial, 2,400 patients were assigned to receive the drug pertuzumab (actually a monoclonal antibody) in addition to standard therapy, while 2,405 patients were assigned to receive standard therapy and placebo. The conclusion was that pertuzumab "significantly improved the rates of invasive-disease-free survival among patients with [a certain kind of] early breast cancer." It may be noted that the trial was sponsored by the manufacturer of the drug, but a commercial interest does not automatically lead to intellectual corruption.

There was no statistically significant difference in the death rates of the two groups at 48 months of follow-up. Thus the drug did not appear to prolong life (though it might be found to have done so on longer follow-up). But results were better when it came to invasive-disease-free survival, which might lead to a better prognosis later. Of those treated with the drug in the most at-risk group of patients (i.e. most likely to have a recurrence), 89.9 percent were free of invasive disease, as against 86.7 percent of those treated with placebo. This result was unlikely to have arisen by chance. One of every 112 people treated with the drug, or one of 56 in the high-risk group, will be spared from invasive disease that would otherwise appear at three years.

The principal side effect of the drug was diarrhea, said to be mainly mild, and lasting only during the treatment itself, for up to a year.[2] It occurred in 9.8 percent of those treated with the drug and 3.7 percent of those who received placebo. Does the benefit of the drug outweigh its disadvantage? Yes, almost certainly. But pertuzumab is probably very expensive (though no price is indicated). Is it worth the cost? That depends on who is paying, and how much. A nasty question.

The other paper that illustrates medical uncertainty concerns the follow-up of patients with early prostate cancer treated either with prostatectomy or by observation (watching and waiting). In general, prostatectomy gave slightly better results as far as mortality was concerned, but the difference was just below statistical significance, which

---

2 Though once again I bear in mind the famous dictum of Sir George Pickering that a minor operation is an operation performed on someone else.

means that there was a slightly greater than 5 percent chance that the results arose by chance. This does not mean, however, that they *did* arise by chance; the superiority of surgery might have been genuine, though not very great. On the other hand, those who underwent surgery experienced more side effects that interfered with their quality of life at two years' follow-up and that persisted at ten years.

The doctor has to advise the patient and the patient has to decide. Science will never by itself eliminate this kind of dilemma, at least not until everyone can remain healthy forever. ◙

July 20, 2017

There were two articles this week that acted as a kind of madeleine for me. They both concern the uncertainty of prognosis at the end of life and the acceptance of death.

The first article, "Managing Uncertainty—Harnessing the Power of Scenario Planning," is really an exercise in what might be called *the higher cliché*. But as Doctor Johnson said, we need more often to be reminded than informed. The main point of the article is that doctors, in offering their prognoses to patients (or their relatives), ought not to confine themselves to bare statistics, such as that there is a 25 percent chance of survival, but give a range of possibilities and explain what those possibilities would be like as subjective experiences.

The article starts with a vignette about an 87-year-old priest who crashes his car and ends up with broken ribs in an intensive care unit. Unable to breathe by himself, he is put on a ventilator. Investigations reveal that he has metastases in his lungs. He has not long to live, though no one can say exactly how long. At first he is highly unrealistic about his own prospects. When told by his surgeon that his risk of death from his injuries at his age is over 90 percent, he feebly scrawls a note asking: "What about my car? When can I drive again?" This shows that he is a man of spirit, but it is virtually certain that he will never drive again; indeed, he might never stand upright again.

The authors say that clinicians often use statistics in an effort to "quantify uncertainty" about outcomes, but those numbers "offer little guidance to patients for managing this uncertainty." Some patients, moreover, may have "blind spots" for the likelihood of a poor outcome, as the elderly priest apparently did. The authors suggest *scenario planning* as a way of discussing uncertainties with patients.

> Scenario planning asks us to accept uncertainty and use it as part of our reasoning. To do so, we must first distinguish irreducible uncertainties from "predetermined elements"—events that have already happened or are likely to occur but whose sequelae have yet to unfold. Identifying these elements promotes insight by highlighting the interaction between forces that drive change and provides an organized way to consider alternative futures.

I am afraid that this kind of thought and prose makes not only my eyes but my whole brain glaze over. It conveys nothing very concrete to me, and nothing very abstract either. Since this kind of prose and thought is now very common in the world, the fault may be with me rather than with it.

The authors use the case of the elderly priest to illustrate what they mean by scenario planning: "The surgeon returned to talk to [the patient] and his family. Still alert and engaged, he listened attentively as she described the best, worst and most likely scenarios for his current care plan." The best case was so bad that the patient asked to be extubated. "He died later that day, surrounded by family."

There seems to me nothing extraordinary about what the surgeon said or did, though I do remember the days when surgeons regarded the continuation of life at all costs as the be-all and end-all of their activity, and did not concern themselves very much with what kind of life it would be. I remember in particular a neurosurgeon who regarded the faint movement of a man's limb as a great triumph after an operation to cure his total paralysis, though he, the neurosurgeon, was not optimistic about the further progress of his patient (who had been a university professor).

My father, who had cancer of the stomach, was offered a palliative operation shortly before he died of it. He was told that it might extend his life by six months; but of those six months, he would spend at least three recovering from the operation—if he ever did recover from it, that is. He turned the operation down; and neither he nor his surgeon, I suspect, had ever heard of *scenario planning*.

The second article reminded me of the death of my mother. It recounts the story of a lady in her eighty-seventh year who had smoked until just over twenty years earlier. She gave up too late, however: by then she had developed emphysema. "She was short of breath walking on a level surface at a modest pace." This was exactly the story of my mother, except that she gave up smoking when she was only forty-eight. I remember perfectly the moment at which I realized that she was suffering from emphysema: I had taken her to Lisbon to celebrate her seventieth birthday, and she had difficulty walking more than a few steps up an incline at a time.

The patient in the article suddenly deteriorated. Her doctors thought that she might just have a condition that they could diagnose and cure, though it was more likely to be incurable and such that would make a return to her previous life impossible. She was content to die undiagnosed.

My mother, at age eighty-five, had an illness from which it was quite unnecessary that she should die. But she estimated that her chances of returning to an independent existence were slight, and she would rather die than live in a dependent way. There were special circumstances in her case, but her wish was respected and no one had to talk of *scenario planning*.

～

Political correctness is like a poison gas that can seep into the most unlikely places. There was a fascinating article in the *Journal* this week titled "Preventing Weight Gain by Blocking Follicle-Stimulating Hormone," part of a series called "Clinical Implications of Basic Research." It reported some experiments on mice, demonstrating that if the action of FSH (a pituitary sex hormone) were blocked by antibodies against it, the mice that were injected with those antibodies developed less fat than those given placebo injections. The subcutaneous, visceral and total fat content of the treated mice was less than that of the untreated mice. "Antibody treatment also increased total energy expenditure," we read, and the effect was "attributed to an increase in resting energy expenditure and not physical activity expenditure."

Of course, it is a far cry from antibody-treated mice to hamburger-consuming humans, yet it is possible that the hormone treatment might be of human application. The authors conclude by saying:

It will be particularly important to assess whether such an antibody [to human FSH] would have fewer off-target effects than other pharmacologic therapies, which have proved to be problematic in the treatment of obesity.

Off-target effects, I presume, means undesired side effects, and seems to me an inferior expression insofar as it might be used to mystify patients, at least for a time. Patients are used to the idea of side effects, but off-target effects will appear to them something different and perhaps less the doctor's fault.

That is not the political correctness to which I referred just above, however. It is actually in a small verbal matter, the very smallness of it demonstrating just how far political correctness has gone. The authors write:

> 3-month old intact female and male C57BL/6J mice were treated for 8 weeks with intraperitoneal injections.... The FSH antibody treatment resulted in significant decreases in fat mass in female and male mice....

In English it would be normal to say "male and female mice" rather than "female and male mice," not because male mice are deemed superior or more important than female mice, but because of the natural rhythm of the language. Euphony requires it, in fact; but obviously this is deemed by someone at the *NEJM* (or possibly the authors themselves) to be of little account by comparison with the chance to strike an ideological blow. The very fact that attention is given to so tiny and arcane a matter is a sign of the determination, thoroughness and fanaticism of those who want to reform language itself, and through it our very souls. Victor Klemperer, a German philologist and diarist of the Nazi era, wrote eloquently of the linguistic distortions practiced by the Nazis; and, of course, the Russian language went through a similar process. Now it seems to be the turn of English, albeit in muted form. ▣

July 27, 2017

Whe n I was a young doctor, I was very proud of having made a
diagnosis of temporal arteritis, now called giant-cell arteritis,
in a man about sixty years old. It was not such good news for him,
of course, for the condition was (and is) a chronic one, with frequent
relapses. The diagnosis was more or less a life sentence. Giant-cell
arteritis is an inflammatory condition of unknown cause that affects the
aortic arch and the extracranial portion of the carotid artery. It causes
a generalized malaise, severe headache, and—if untreated—blindness
and stroke.

The only treatment available then, and for long afterward, was steroids. Relapses required further dosages, reduced or increased according
to the results of blood tests for inflammation. Unfortunately, steroids are
not themselves without many side effects, including very severe ones,
especially when taken for a long time and in large doses.

This week's *Journal* reports the results of a trial that gives some
hope of more prolonged relief to sufferers and is an example of what
seems to me an increasingly rare genre, an unequivocal success. It was
a trial of tocilizumab, an inhibitor of one of the substances produced
by cells of the body itself that are thought to provoke the disease. In
the trial, 250 patients with the disease were divided into four groups,
the first consisting of 100 patients and the other three of 50 each. The
first two groups were given injections of tocilizumab either weekly or
every other week, in addition to the usual treatment of steroids in a
26-week program of tapering the dose; the other two groups received

placebo injections along with the usual treatment in either a 26- or a 52-week program of tapering the dose. The physicians administering the steroids did not know whether the patients had been given tocilizumab or placebo.

For once, there was no doubt about the results, as measured both by the percentage of patients with sustained remission and by the amount of steroids the patients had to be given according to the activity of the disease. Just over half of both groups of patients treated with tocilizumab and steroids had prolonged remission, whereas only 16 percent of patients give placebo and steroids experienced such remission. Moreover, those in the placebo groups needed nearly twice as much steroid supplementation as the groups treated with tocilizumab. Furthermore, and unusually, the side-effect profile was better in the treatment groups than in the placebo groups, possibly because of the higher doses of steroids that the latter required to control their symptoms. No patient died during the trial period of a year.

These results were excellent, at least by comparison with all previous treatment—which, of course, is the proper standard of comparison.[1] They fall far short of perfection, of course: only half the patients responded positively to the drug, and no one knows whether the effect will last beyond a year, or indeed what the long-term adverse effects might be. But for the moment they are a triumph, and a herald of better things to come, insofar as they are the result of the application of basic research and not merely the result of serendipity, as so many medical advances have been.

The trial was financed by the pharmaceutical company that manufactures tocilizumab. The paper states:

> The investigators and sponsor [i.e. the pharmaceutical company] designed the trial and gathered and analyzed the data. The sponsor

---

1 In politics, people are apt to compare the present not with what has gone before, but with an ideal normal that has never existed, and probably never could exist. Thus, if you tell people that enormous numbers of Indians have been lifted out of abject poverty in India, a fair proportion will respond by saying that nevertheless there is still much poverty in the countryside. So there is: but there has never been a case in the whole history of the world in which people were lifted equally, simultaneously and massively from poverty.

provided tocilizumab and placebo and participated in the writing and editing of the drafts of the manuscript. ...All the authors [sixteen of them] participated in the writing of every draft of the manuscript, with the assistance of medical writers paid by the sponsor.

This would be enough to raise the suspicions of those who imagine that *any* involvement of the pharmaceutical industry in medical research must be corrupting, and certainly the payment of professional "medical writers" has been the object of much criticism in the past. Their job is to put a spin on things without actually lying (whereas politicians put a spin on things *and* lie). But I find it hard to believe that these results—which in fact are consonant with other findings—have been manufactured out of whole cloth and are but the manipulations of a company trying to sell its fantastically expensive new drug.

Those who are inclined to see the corruption of commerce everywhere are far less inclined to discern the self-interest of governmental and quasi-governmental organizations. It is as if the mere fact of being paid from public funds renders people honest and totally without personal interests, as if the receipt of a government salary were sufficient to turn those who receive it into a philosopher-king à la Plato.

In this same issue of the *Journal* is a "Special Report" by two high officials of the National Institute on Drug Abuse in Washington, D.C. At the end of the article, titled "The Role of Science in Addressing the Opioid Crisis," is the following declaration: "No conflict of interest relevant to this article was reported." Not to accuse anyone of anything, but this is surely very naive.[2]

The National Institute on Drug Abuse receives funds on the promise that purely biomedical research will solve, or at any rate vastly ameliorate, the problem of drug abuse in society. If this promise were to prove illusory, the funds would dry up and those employed by the

2 The authors also tell us: "We thank... Walter Koroshetz, Linda Porter, and David Thomas for their analyses on the NIH's [National Institutes of Health's] pain research portfolio and priorities." *Portfolio* is surely an odd word to use in the case of a staff and institution without personal or sectional interests. It is a word I expect to hear from the mouth of my financial adviser.

Institute would presumably lose their jobs. Indeed, the Institute first defined addiction as a brain disease not because it was a scientifically established fact, but because Congress, its paymaster, would stump up for the promise of a purely technical solution to a purely technical problem, but not for a much more nuanced approach. What starts as a convenient lie ends up, when repeated often enough, as a convenient truth.

Thus, in an echo of what Congress was told more than forty years ago, we read: "Opioid addiction...is a chronic, relapsing illness." Furthermore: "Abundant research has shown that sustained treatment over years or even a lifetime is often necessary to achieve and maintain long-term recovery."

This is a partial way of putting it, to say the least. What experience has shown is that *no* sustained treatment, indeed hardly any treatment of any kind, is necessary for whole populations to abandon their opioid drugs—for example, in China when Mao Zedong took the short way with addicts, or in the United States when thousands of soldiers returned from their tours of duty in the Vietnam War addicted to heroin and then gave it up without assistance. These examples cast doubt not only on the assertion that lifelong treatment is often necessary to obtain long-term abstinence, but also on the concept of addiction as an illness of the same ilk as, say, Parkinson's disease. The article partakes of the oldest rhetorical tricks in the book: *suggestio falsi* and *suppressio veri*.

Given the scale of the epidemic of deaths from opioid overdoses in the United States (more than 30,000 a year at current rates), no one with a sense of irony, let alone humor, could have written the following: "In the past few decades, we have made remarkable strides in our understanding of the biologic mechanisms that underlie pain and addiction." With a little more such progress (and more funding, of course), perhaps we could get the figure up to 100,000 a year, to which the only solution would be—yes, you guessed it—more funding for the National Institute on Drug Abuse. ▪

August 3, 2017

The statistical way of thinking has entered deeply into my soul, so to speak. Thus, when someone makes a statement such as "an exceptional number of doctors have been good writers," I immediately ask myself, and often the person who has made the statement, "How many doctors would you expect to have been good writers?" In other words, what is the rule to which the number is an exception? I was musing one day with a bookseller of my acquaintance over the fact—if it is a fact—of the surprisingly large number of doctor-writers, when he asked, "How many dentist-writers do you know?" While there is approximately one dentist for every five doctors, it is obvious that there are many more than five times as many doctor-writers as dentist-writers. There might be fewer dentist-writers than one would *expect*, while doctors are merely filling their quota.

Similarly, if someone says that our criminal justice system is bad because there have been too many miscarriages of justice (in the direction of wrongful conviction, of course), I ask, "How many miscarriages of justice would you expect?" A perfect human institution is almost inconceivable, after all. And that applies to medical practice: it will never be free of error.

In the interest of minimizing medical errors, most doctors trust the properly controlled double-blind trial, and indeed now believe it to be almost the only scientific evidence there can be in favor of medical treatment. An essay in this week's *Journal* points out that this is far from the case. In fact, a moment's reflection on the history of medicine should have been sufficient to tell us this, but in a busy life doctors don't have time for moments of reflection. They, like everybody else, are subject to intellectual fashion. We are often more like religious converts than rational beings.

It was only comparatively recently that doctors came to realize that their personal experience, or that of others in authority, was not always sufficient to prove that a medical treatment or technique actually worked. This realization led in due course to an overestimation of the importance and the reliability of controlled trials. After all, no one really needed a controlled trial to know that anesthetics work. (Incidentally, the use of anesthetics spread as quickly in the late 1840s as any new technique today, and possibly faster.)

The essay lays out the reasons why double-blind controlled trials have their pitfalls as well as their advantages, and are not a panacea for medical ignorance. For one thing, such trials are conducted on highly selected patients of a kind rarely encountered in daily practice. Then too, the behavior of patients during the course of such trials may be very different from that of patients in everyday circumstances, particularly with regard to compliance, the degree to which they take the treatment as prescribed. A drug may have a wonderful effect during a trial, but it will be of little use if people fail to take it—as is all too often the case.

Another weakness or defect (if you prefer stronger language) is that there are many questions that such trials cannot answer. If the dose or doses chosen for the trial are wrong, the results will be wrong. The results are valid only for patients similar in all respects to those chosen for the trial, and only for the periods of time the trial lasts. If a medication works over a period of three months, it does not follow therefrom that it will work over a period of twelve months, or ten years. Moreover, side effects, sometimes serious, may manifest themselves only after a long delay. Controlled trials will not show this. And some forms of treatment might not lend themselves very easily to controlled trials, for logistical reasons. Numbers unmanageable in size may be needed to demonstrate an effect, and the larger the numbers, the more difficult it is to be sure that the protocols of the trial have been complied with.

There are many other sources of scientific evidence in medicine than the controlled trial, and yet many of us doctors cling to it as what we call the "gold standard" of medical evidence. (I leave it to economists to decide whether the gold standard was a good or a bad thing, by whatever standards of evidence they, the economists, use.) Doctors, like everyone else, are not immune from the desire that there should be a panacea, whether for illness or for ignorance.

Now that American doctors have finally woken up to the epidemic of opioid addiction for which they are partly responsible, they are searching for alternatives to prescribe for chronic pain. They have fixed on a group of drugs called the gabapentinoids, whose use (or should I say misuse?) is ascending vertiginously.

These drugs have not been shown—by double-blind controlled trials, which would be just the ticket in the circumstances—to work in most of the conditions for which doctors are now prescribing them. It is almost a replay of what went before with opioids. According to an article in the *Journal* this week, both gabapentin and pregabalin are being diverted by people prescribed them on to a black market. Prescriptions of pregabalin have more than doubled in the last four years, undoubtedly to the great delight of the pharmaceutical company that manufactures it. In fact, the company has already paid a fine for mis-selling the drug to doctors, but as Mobutu Sese Seko said, it takes two to be corrupt.

The drugs, though almost certainly useless or only very marginally useful in the conditions for which they are being prescribed, are not without side effects, particularly neurological ones. They cause sedation and dizziness, and it is probable (though the article does not mention it specifically) that many people drive under their influence. One statistic mentioned in the article caught my attention, referring to a trial in which pregabalin was shown to be not of value in the treatment of sciatica (for which it is nonetheless frequently prescribed): "In the sciatica trial, 40% of patients taking pregabalin reported dizziness, as compared with 13% of those taking placebo." That 13 percent of patients taking a placebo should experience dizziness is surely remarkable: for example, *no* patients in a double-blind placebo-controlled trial of a drug for treatment of acute myeloid leukemia reported suffering from dizziness.

This suggests, I think, a different psychology in those with pain from sciatica; and it is interesting that the authors of the article say:

"Indiscriminate…use of gabapentinoids reinforces the tendency to view the treatment of pain through a pharmaceutical lens…." In other words, these new drugs may perpetuate the inclination to treat chronic pain merely by pills, even when such pain has been shown to be much more closely related to the patient's psychosocial state than to his physical condition.

This seems to show that nothing durable has been learned by the medical profession from the opioid epidemic. Experience is one of the many things from which we do not learn.

～

There is a rather chilling letter from the Netherlands at the back of the *Journal*, titled "End-of-Life Decisions in the Netherlands over 25 Years." The authors conducted a survey of doctors about the numbers they assisted to die, or outright killed, over the period from 1990 to 2015. No more than 78 percent of doctors surveyed answered, which gives plenty of scope for the other 22 percent to have flouted the law by deciding for themselves, without reference to the law's constraints, who should live and who should die.

In any case, by the report of those doctors who answered the survey, the percentage of deaths by euthanasia rose in that period from 1.7 percent in 1990 to 4.5 percent in 2015. About 8.3 percent of those who died in 2015 had requested being put down, the request not being granted in 3.8 percent. But here is a little statistic that one might have thought would interest the police: "Ending of life without an explicit patient request decreased, from 0.8% to 0.3%." In other words, doctors were outright murdering their patients, just not so often as before. Whom were the doctors assisting to die? The letter informs us:

> In 2015, the percentage of patients who were older than 80 years was higher than in 1990 (35% vs. 22%), as was the percentage of patients who had an estimated life expectancy of more than a month (27% vs. 16%).

We learn also that in 2015, "92% of the patients who received physician assisted dying had a serious somatic disease." This means, of course, that 8 percent did not. Moreover, a "serious somatic disease" is not quite the same as a disease that will kill you in short order.

The last sentence of the letter says that assisted dying in the Netherlands "is provided predominantly to patients with severe disease but increasingly involves older patients and those with a life expectancy of more than a month." One of the principal objections to assisted suicide and outright euthanasia is that it is the beginning of a slippery slope. Does this survey provide evidence that the slope is indeed being slipped down, at least in the Netherlands? ▣

August 10, 2017

An objection to pharmaceutical industry overinvolvement in medical research is that it biases or distorts results in its own favor. I leave it to others to decide whether alternative means of funding research would be better, or possible. But I could not help wondering whether the report on a trial of a drug in a certain kind of breast cancer, "Olaparib for Metastatic Breast Cancer in Patients with a Germline BRCA Mutation," was perhaps overoptimistic in its conclusions in the abstract at the head of the article:

> Olaparib monotherapy provided a significant benefit over standard therapy; median progression-free survival was 2.8 months longer and the risk of disease progression or death was 42% lower with olaparib monotherapy than with standard therapy.

I thought there might be yet another dog that did not bark within the body of the article, where we learn:

> The trial was designed in collaboration between the principal investigator and AstraZeneca [a giant pharmaceutical company]. AstraZeneca was responsible for overseeing the collection, analysis and interpretation of the data. An external independent data and safety monitoring committee performed two interim reviews of the safety data. The manuscript was written with medical-writing support, which was funded by AstraZeneca.

The independent monitoring committee, then, appears to have had oversight *only* of the safety data, and not of the data related to the other results of the trial. (Was this possibly a paranoid overreaction on my part?)

Be that as it may, according to a graph in the article, 70 percent of the patients were dead 24 months later in both the experimental group and the control group, and overall survival was barely distinguishable between the two even up to that point. In this light, a superior progression-free survival of 2.8 months without much improvement in survival seems to belie the optimistic tone of the conclusion, and might potentially be misleading of those doctors (probably the great majority) who read only the abstracts of papers. The word "significant" in this context is an ambiguous one, because it could mean either statistically significant or clinically significant (or both); and although the authors attempt to provide evidence that the results were clinically significant, for the patients themselves, the test of clinical significance was a matter of judging the differences in the responses that patients gave on questionnaires about quality of life to be significant. It felt like entering a hall of mirrors.

This is not to say that olaparib does not represent an advance in the treatment of this type of breast cancer. Great leaps forward occur in medicine, but so too do accretions of small steps forward. But contrary to popular conception, scientific papers, at least in the medical field, often are not self-interpreting and yield different meanings according to the initial point of view of the reader.

An article titled "Supporting Women's Autonomy in Prenatal Testing" is written by a lawyer, a physician and a doctor of philosophy, and comes from a hospital and its bioethics department and an institute of bioethics. I have to admit to a visceral mistrust and even an unfounded prejudice against bioethicists, but the plain fact is that new technology inevitably throws up new ethical dilemmas that must be resolved somehow, even when they are not really resolvable. But I fear the kind of person who, from premises that seem to him reasonable and with logic that seems to him impeccable, comes to an obviously revolting conclusion, yet prefers to believe that conclusion rather than doubt either his premises or his reasoning. A philosopher might be defined as a man who overestimates the importance of intellectual consistency in practical matters.

Patient autonomy is the philosopher's stone of modern medical ethics, or perhaps I should say the elixir of medical correctness. The present article uses it in connection with the ethical problems posed by prenatal genetic testing.

It will be possible before long to examine the entire genome of a fetus prenatally. However, the interpretation or meaning of the results will often be ambiguous, where it is not completely unknown. Furthermore, the ambiguity will never be resolved: it is inherent in the information, because many conditions with a genetic predisposition are not simply and monocausally genetic in origin. A fetus might have the genes that give it a tendency to a disease (either soon or late in life), but this information by itself cannot tell anyone whether a person will ever actually suffer from the disease, or even give an approximate likelihood. It depends on many other factors. Moreover, even where we think we know that a certain genetic defect causes a disease, our knowledge may turn out to be false, as the authors illustrate with an example.

They point out that more information is not by itself necessarily a good thing, especially where its meaning or significance is equivocal. They write:

> Two recent studies suggest that people's desire for genomic information in the prenatal context varies. In a study of pregnant women receiving abnormal prenatal chromosome microarray results, Barbara Bernhardt and colleagues found that although many women saw the offer of more information about their fetus as "too good to pass up," they were blindsided by the results. Many of the women who received uninterpretable or uncertain results viewed them as "toxic knowledge" that they wished they did not have. The researchers therefore called for "a thorough discussion of the various uncertainties with abnormal [testing] results" as part of pretest counseling.

Thomas Gray was right a quarter of a millennium ago when, without elaborate study but with the employment of mere common sense, he wondered if people really needed to "know their fate," for happiness flies swiftly, and "where ignorance is bliss, 'Tis folly to be wise."

It is surely common sense that, before a test is performed, both the doctor performing it and the patient should understand the significance of the possible results, and the difference that the knowledge will make. But is there a right to ignorance, as much as a right to knowledge? Consider the example of Huntington's chorea, a neuro-degenerative disease causing involuntary movements, psychiatric disturbances, dementia and death. Fifty percent of children with a parent who has Huntington's chorea will inherit the disease, and it can now be predicted with certainty whether or not they will develop it by a simple blood test.[1] Unfortunately, in hereditary cases, those who carry it may have children before the disease manifests itself, and there might also be grandchildren at risk of developing it from an index case before anyone is aware of it. Suppose the parent does not want to know but the grandchild does: whose right—to ignorance or to knowledge—trumps whose?

In a discussion of decision making with regard to offspring, there is a conspicuous absence, namely, the figure of the father. Indeed, the very word *father* does not appear in the article, as if reproduction were by parthenogenesis and no man need be involved. The family is mentioned once, but only in the context of the difficulties it faces when a handicapped child is born:

> Policies in a range of areas, from education to social care, that support people with disabilities and their families are also needed so that women's choices are less likely to be constrained by financial concerns or fears for the future welfare of the disabled child.

What is most important for the authors is the autonomy of women, respect for which, they say, "crucially requires access to abortion services."

In the authors' world, then, women not only do but ought to float free in a complete social vacuum (apart from social security). No doubt this is an approximation of how some women live, but the results are happy for no one. ▪

---

1 Not all cases of Huntington's chorea are inherited. Some arise by spontaneous mutation of the gene involved in its causation.

August 17, 2017

The expression *alternative facts*, the use of which is a kind of short-hand for all that is wrong with the current American administration, has never seemed to me quite so absurd as is sometimes alleged. If I say that the First World War was caused by X, basing my opinion on facts a, b and c, you can say, quite reasonably, "I don't agree, it was caused by Y," and base your argument on facts d, e and f. Your facts are alternative to the ones that I have adduced, but if they are facts they are part of the truth. We differ, of course, in our assessment of the significance of the two sets of facts, but this difference does not make either of them lies. Deliberate untruths, on the other hand, are not alternative facts, but lies.

An article in the *NEJM* titled "Medical Education in the Era of Alternative Facts" made my heart sink, as I thought it would be a festival or compendium of political correctness. So I was pleasantly surprised to find that, to the contrary, it was eminently sensible (and therefore, perhaps, a little dull). The surprise was pleasant in part because it reassured me that my mind, if not open exactly, was at least ajar.

The author, a teacher at Virginia Commonwealth University, under-estimates somewhat the need for medical students to learn current medical dogma as if it were indubitable fact. After all, doctors are practical people, having to act more often than to reflect—to be more often Don Quixote than Hamlet. It is certainly desirable, as he says, that they should have inquiring minds and an openness to new hypotheses, for science is not so much a body of settled fact as a way of approaching reality.

But the degree to which science recognizes no settled facts can be exaggerated. When the author says that we live at a time when "uncomfortable facts are derided as 'fake news' while fabrications masquerade as reality," he does not point his finger in any particular political direction, for the suppression of truth and the suggestion of falsehood are permanent temptations of anyone engaged upon matters of dispute.

The author says one thing that particularly struck a chord with me: "Critical review" of scientific literature, he writes, "is such an essential skill that I believe it should be taught, practiced, and honed throughout all 4 years of medical school and even formally in postgraduate education." This book, as I mentioned in the introduction, was partly prompted by the difficulty that my nephew Joseph had with a medical school examination in precisely this skill: how to read a scientific paper. After failing the exam on the first try, he asked for my help in preparing to retake it. He had been given a paper to read and assess—from the *New England Journal of Medicine*, as it happens—about some alleged statistical association (between drinking coffee and cancer of the pancreas, I think it was). Before my tuition, he could see nothing wrong with it; afterward, he said with joyful surprise, *"Mais c'est nul, cet article!"* (But it's worthless, this article!) Whether or not my assistance had anything to do with it, he passed on the second attempt.

I had given him a few simple rules to follow, including the criteria to assess whether a statistical association implied a causative relationship. I have never been much of a teacher, but I can see how teaching can act as a feather duster of the mind.

Using my own rules, I evaluated a paper in the *Journal* on a trial of low-dose aspirin in the prevention of preterm preeclampsia[1] compared with placebo. Does aspirin work?

In summary, the answer is yes. Of 798 mothers deemed at risk for preeclampsia who took aspirin (or rather who were assigned to the aspirin group, and who mostly complied with the treatment), 1.6 percent developed preeclampsia. Of 822 mothers who were given placebo, 4.3

---

1 Preeclampsia is the development of high blood pressure and proteinuria during pregnancy. It leads to worse outcomes, and when it becomes severe it can be dangerous and even fatal for the mother.

percent developed preeclampsia. The difference in the ratio was very unlikely to have arisen by chance. The authors conclude, quite justly:

> This randomized trial showed that among women with singleton [i.e. not twin] pregnancies who were identified by means of first-trimester screening as being at high risk for preterm preeclampsia, the administration of aspirin at a dose of 150 mg per day from 11 to 14 weeks of gestation until 36 weeks of gestation resulted in a significantly lower incidence of preterm preeclampsia than that with placebo.

How important an advance in knowledge, from the point of view of the practitioner, is this paper written by twenty authors? It is rather difficult to say. In order to find the 1,620 mothers who took part in the trial, 26,941 had first to be screened. Of these, 2,641 were found to be at risk of developing preeclampsia, but 865 of them declined to participate in the trial, and of the 1,776 who accepted initially, 152 withdrew and four were lost to follow-up.

Aspirin is very cheap, which is a great advantage. Even so, it is known that adherence to a regime is considerably greater during the conduct of a trial than in normal practice. Moreover, preventing preeclampsia is not an end in itself unless doing so conduces to some other good, such as healthier mothers or children. One is, after all, treating a person and not a blood pressure.

The trial did not show any *statistically significant* benefit for the mothers of children: there was no *statistically significant* decrease in stillbirths, for example, or need for blood transfusion. There was no *statistically significant* decrease in the rate of miscarriage. Nor was there such a decrease in low birth weight or (alternatively) in high birth weight. Most of the differences pointed in the same direction, to the advantage of aspirin over placebo. The problem was that the difference was not large enough to reach statistical significance with this size of sample. If the sample size had been larger, the differences might well (and probably *would*, I think) have reached statistical significance.[2]

---

2 A statistically significant difference between two groups is, by convention, a difference that has a less than one in twenty likelihood of having arisen by chance. A statistically significant difference need not be significant in other ways, e.g. clinically. This is often forgotten.

If this were the only paper that a busy practitioner read on this subject (by no means the first, and certainly not the last, to be written), would he prescribe aspirin for patients at risk of preeclampsia? I certainly would, perhaps as much to avoid trouble for myself if I failed to do so, as for their benefit.

The opening paragraph of this paper illustrates one of the common difficulties in the interpretation of medical papers.

> Preeclampsia is an important cause of death and complications for the mother and baby. The risk of such complications is considerably higher when the disease is severe and of early onset, leading to pre-term birth at less than 37 weeks of gestation.

This is all perfectly true, but it might be perfectly true even when the risk is so small as not to be worth worrying about. Doubling or trebling a tiny risk may still mean that the risk is tiny; and reducing that tiny risk by half might require treating an enormous number of people. Again, it would be helpful to have the absolute as well as relative risks to hand, since busy doctors will probably not work them out from the figures given. Where the absolute risk is not provided, one has the suspicion, perhaps not always justified, that what is being said is trivial.

In other words, what we need are alternative facts. ◼

August 24, 2017

When I was at school, we had a boy in our class whom we all envied. He suffered from rheumatic heart disease, which excused him from the athletic activities in the winter cold that we detested but which the masters insisted were good for our character. In addition, acute exacerbations meant that he could be off school for several weeks at a time, enjoying the luxurious pleasures of continual bed rest. At that time in our lives, the prospect of a greatly reduced life expectancy, the need for heart surgery, and an early death after years of suffering did not impinge much, if at all, upon our consciousness. The immediate privileges of the ill were what caught our imagination.

Practically no child in a developed country nowadays would suffer from rheumatic fever and the consequent heart disease. The disease has been almost as thoroughly eradicated as polio; and while students at medical school in my day spent much time learning about the disease and its cardiac sequelae, it has now almost disappeared from the curriculum, as the authors of an editorial in the *Journal* point out:

> During their training, medical students in developed countries rarely, if ever, see a child with acute rheumatic fever, and questions about rheumatic heart disease have largely disappeared from licensing examinations.

But just as reports of Mark Twain's death were greatly exaggerated, so the belief that rheumatic fever and rheumatic heart disease are no more is an exaggeration—though one based upon a partial truth. Whether the exaggeration or the partial truth is the more important is perhaps a matter of taste and Weltanschauung.

A paper titled "Global, Regional, and National Burden of Rheumatic Heart Disease, 1990–2015" traces the evolution of the disease in the last quarter century. It can hardly be a matter of much consolation for those suffering from the disease that the overall annual death rate from it in the world (if the authors' calculations are to be trusted) has nearly halved in that period, from 9.2 deaths per 100,000 to 4.8 deaths per 100,000. The absolute number of deaths has remained more or less the same, but of course in the meantime the population of the world has greatly increased.

Interestingly, though not remarked in the paper, is the fact that the reduction of rheumatic heart disease is evidence that the world is becoming more equal. The article explains at the beginning that the disease "is a sequela of acute rheumatic fever, which is usually a disease of poverty associated with overcrowding, poor sanitation, and other social determinants of poor health." By 1990, rheumatic heart disease had already declined so much in developed countries that it had ceased to be an important subject in medical schools. This means that the decline in the death rate from rheumatic heart disease in subsequent years took place disproportionately in the poorer parts of the world, where the disease is now mostly concentrated: 73 percent of the cases of rheumatic heart disease in 2015 were in India, China, Pakistan and the Congo. There were twenty countries in which the disease appeared in more than 1 percent of the population of an age to have it. Nevertheless, global inequality in this respect has been shrinking.

I think it unlikely that the authors would have refrained from animadverting on an increase of inequality if they had found that the death rate from rheumatic heart disease was rising in the poorer parts of the world. Decreasing inequality is, paradoxically, less gratifying to people in favor of equality (as I assume are most of the authors), because often it has occurred spontaneously, without their express intervention or direction. It is an indication that their role is not as providential as perhaps they would have liked. Moreover, it was not the desire to be more equal but the desire to be richer that fueled the growth in wealth on a mass scale in the two most populous countries in the world, India and

China, which together accounted for 60 percent of cases of rheumatic heart disease in the world in 2015. The decline in the rate of mortality from that disease in those two countries is a sign of their accelerating ascent.

In a study of this kind, a great deal depends on sophisticated statistical calculation which I cannot pretend to understand and which I doubt that more than a tiny percentage of the medical profession understands. We have therefore to take both the bona fides and the competence of the authors on faith, and assume that the editors have conscientiously performed their task of weeding out the grosser forms of error. But a wonderful phrase caught my eye in a passage that describes the authors' methods of statistical analysis of their data:

> All data were analyzed with the use of a Bayesian mixed-effects meta-regression tool (designated DisMod-MR 2.1) that was developed for the Global Burden of Disease study. DisMod-MR 2.1 is a compartmental model that consists of three states—susceptible, diseased, and dead—with state transitions determined by the rates of incidence, remission, excess mortality and other cause mortality.

As a summary of human life, the three-compartmental model could hardly be bettered or more succinct: we are all either susceptible or diseased or dead. No human being has ever existed who does not fall into one of those three categories.

John Donne put it somewhat more lengthily but certainly more poetically four centuries ago:

> Variable, and therefore miserable condition of man! this minute I was well, and am ill, this minute. I am surprised with a sudden change, and alteration to worse, and can impute it to no cause, nor call it by any name. We study health, and we deliberate upon our meats, and drink, and air, and exercises, and we hew and we polish every stone that goes to that building; and so our health is a long and a regular work: but in a minute a cannon batters all, overthrows all, demolishes all; a sickness unprevented for all our diligence, unsuspected for all our curiosity; nay, undeserved, if we consider only disorder, summons us, seizes us, possesses us, destroys us in an instant.

Rheumatic fever and associated heart disease does not surprise by sudden change, however; it slowly prepares a man for death and incapacitates him over many years. It is even now responsible for nearly a third of a million deaths each year, perhaps many more according to the editorial that accompanies the research article, for the authors of the editorial claim that for every case of rheumatic heart disease that is detected clinically, there are three to ten cases that remain undetected.

The authors of the editorial point out what they think is an anomaly in the funding of research into various diseases. Tuberculosis, AIDS and malaria each are responsible for three to five times as many deaths as rheumatic heart disease, but attract five hundred to a thousand times more money for research. "It would seem timely," say the authors, "for scientific investigation, media interest and research [into rheumatic fever and heart disease] to be resurrected." According to the table provided, $559,000,000 was devoted to TB research worldwide in 2013, while rheumatic fever got only $900,000, which amounts to virtually nothing and indicates a near-complete loss of scientific interest. Perhaps this is because the epidemiological conditions propitious for the spread of this disease have been known for many years, and the causative organism, *Streptococcus* A, has never been shown to be resistant to penicillin. Therefore the means by which the disease may be eliminated are already more or less settled: better social conditions and the prompt treatment of streptococcal sore throat with penicillin. The rapid decline of the disease suggests that a kind of pincer movement on it is already occurring. Its days are numbered.

The authors of the editorial try to persuade us otherwise. Even now, they write, "occasional outbreaks of rheumatic heart disease have been reported in recent decades...in the United States." This is not entirely convincing, since the outbreak they cite in support of their assertion took place in 1987. For me, the greatest remaining mystery of the disease is a phenomenon called Sydenham's chorea (also known as St. Vitus's dance), first described by Thomas Sydenham in the seventeenth century. This is a condition in which children who suffer from streptococcal sore throat (a precursor to rheumatic fever) later develop uncontrolled, undirected movements and even late psychological changes such as obsessive-compulsive disorder. This, surely, is worthy of intense research, irrespective of how many people are concerned. ▣

August 31, 2017

If he were alive today, Pontius Pilate would ask "What is equity?"— and would not stay for an answer. Perhaps he would be right, for what is equitable, or fair, is by no means easy to determine.

The first article in this week's *Journal* bears the title "A Tale of Two Epidemics—HCV Treatment among Native Americans and Veterans." HCV is hepatitis C virus, an infection that affects principally the liver and leads in about 30 percent of cases to cirrhosis and, in a smaller number, to cancer of the liver. Almost alone of all viral infections it can be cured, though with drugs that, at least for the moment, are very expensive: a full three-month course costs about $80,000. It is unlikely that many of the sufferers can pay for the drugs themselves.

It will perhaps not surprise readers to learn that American veterans with HCV—nearly 200,000 of them—have much better access to treatment than do American Indians, who have the highest mortality of any group of people in North America. Their death rate is 12.95 per 100,000, compared with 4.95 for the population as a whole.

Interestingly (but not remarked upon in the article), a graph shows that the incidence of new HCV infections among whites in the United States began a fairly steep rise in about 2010, something not seen in other races except American Indians. The rate among whites is now nearly four times higher than among blacks and ten times higher than among "Asians or Pacific Islanders": Chinese, Indian, Vietnamese, Samoans and others, lumped together as one race, which might not please all of them.

The great majority of new cases of infection with HCV are attributable to intravenous drug abuse (or "use," as the *Journal* now seems to insist upon calling it). One of the former means of transmission, by contaminated blood in transfusions, has been overcome by screening donated blood for the virus. Sexual transmission is rare, as is transmission by contaminated needles or ink in tattoo parlors.

What, then, does this increase among whites in America mean or signify? According to a paper from 2012 titled "Hepatitis C Virus in American Indian/Alaskan Native and Aboriginal Peoples of North America," in the journal *Viruses*, "Liver diseases, such as hepatitis C (HCV), are 'broken spirit' diseases." This term is not defined further, but the authors, both of them hepatologists, state that "broken spirit" diseases "encompass alcoholic induced liver disease, hepatitis C virus (HCV) and hepatitis B virus (HBV),[1] along with the rise of non-alcoholic induced fatty liver disease (NAFLD) and non-alcoholic steatohepatitis (NASH)."[2]

The usage *"broken spirit" diseases* is ambiguous, perhaps deliberately so. It could mean diseases occasioned by a broken spirit, or it could mean diseases that cause a broken spirit. The former is the only meaning that really makes sense: a broken spirit causes people to drink or eat too much, or inject themselves with drugs. The authors of this paper were writing at a time when treatment was not as effective as it would become by 2017 (five years can be a long time in the history of therapeutics), and they therefore concluded that:

> Although new therapies for HCV infection offer hope, prevention should be a priority. In prevention and treatment it is necessary that historical and personal trauma be addressed as they are crucial to the etiology of high risk behaviors that drive HCV infection and other broken spirit diseases.

Are we to suppose, then, that the rise of HCV among white Americans is a manifestation of a broken spirit, and if so, what is it that broke it? Could their "historical and personal trauma" perhaps be an

---

1 Also spread predominantly by intravenous drug abuse.

2 The most common cause of both NAFLD and NASH is thought to be obesity.

increasing realization that their racial hegemony in the United States is in decline? Meanwhile, the situation of black Americans improved dramatically: according to the graph in the *NEJM* article, their rate of HCV infection in the year 2000 was at least twice that of whites, but by 2015 it was just over a quarter. Other sources, however, suggest that the situation of blacks relative to whites with regard to HCV may not have improved.

The white population of the United States is, of course, a very large one, susceptible to disaggregation according to criteria other than race. And even in those portions of the larger population in which the rate of infection is high relatively speaking, it is still low in absolute terms. New cases of HCV among American Indians, who have the highest rate of any group, run at 1.8 per 100,000 per year, and among whites, at 0.9 per 100,000 per year. If, as is plausible, people take to "high risk behaviors" because of historical traumas, they take to them very unequally on an individual basis. The majority of people do not take to them, even in the most unfavorable of circumstances.

As is so often the case nowadays, there is a certain unctuousness that runs through the *NEJM* article, or at least I find it so. The replacement of the word *abuse* by *use* in connection with taking heroin illicitly, for example, arises not from the belief that taking heroin for nonmedical reasons is not (as previously thought) a bad thing to do, but from the desire to avoid being seen as illiberal and censorious. At the same time, the person who calls it *use* rather than *abuse* will, for the same reason, subscribe to the modern orthodoxy that addiction to heroin is a disease like any other. These mental contortions are a symptom of a wish to be thought good, in a society in which being good is increasingly a matter of holding the right opinions and using "correct" language.

The article ends with impeccably correct opinion on "disparities" in the treatment of HCV infection:

> The U.S. government has a special responsibility to both American Indians and veterans. Veterans have served their country. Indian Nations, after a long struggle, have treaties ratified by the government that dictate sovereign nation-to-nation relationships and a federal trust responsibility to uphold treaty agreements. The current disparities in HCV resources and mortality give the appearance of neglect

at best—and institutional racism at worst. American Indian nations deserve the same quality of care and the same level of resources as the VA.

But do they? On what grounds is everyone's desert equal? The veterans have served their country; the Indians have treaties. Sovereign nation-to-nation relationships do not usually include responsibility for the health care of one of the parties to the relationship; indeed, sovereignty more or less precludes such a responsibility. Being sovereign means being responsible for what goes on in a certain territory. Assistance may be sought from outside by the sovereign power, but it is granted as a matter of discretion, not of right. If the United States owes a duty of care to the Indians—as surely most people would say that it does— then the treaties are not sovereign nation-to-nation covenants, but something else.

HCV disease is the consequence of high-risk behavior that must, at least to a considerable extent, be under the control of the individual. I do not see the equity in making others pay for the deleterious consequences of voluntary conduct; but it is at least arguable that the veterans, who have served their country, have done something more to *deserve* the care that they receive afterward.

"So," I hear people say in my mind's ear, "you think it is a good thing that American Indians should die of an essentially curable disease?" Of course I do not; I am concerned only to point out that the arguments employed in this article seem to me to be false. If one desires to do something about HCV among American Indians, it is from a sense of charity, not from desert. But this would no doubt be regarded as paternalistic, and paternalism is as much to be avoided (for those who wish to keep caste with a certain ilk of which they believe themselves members) as is the word *abuse* to describe a habit of injecting oneself with medically unprescribed heroin.

I do not pretend to have the solution to the admitted tragedy of the American Indian (or the Australian Aborigine); but I think Pascal was right when he said:

> All our dignity consists in thought. It is by this that we must raise ourselves up.... Let us work, therefore, to think well: for such is the principle of morality. ∎

September 6, 2017

Although most health-care systems in the developed world do the majority of what they are supposed to do, anxiety about them is, if not quite universal, at least very common. Nowhere is this more so than in the United States, which spends far more per capita on health care than any other country in the world, but does not seem to get the best results.

The first article this week is titled "From Last to First—Could the U.S. Health Care System Become the Best in the World?" The title implies that the American health-care system as presently constituted is the worst in the world—the word *world* being here used in a technical rather than a literal sense, for not even its fiercest critic would claim that it was worse than the health-care system of, say, Burkina Faso or the Central African Republic.

The deficiencies of the American system are considerable. Half-socialized and half-private—the latter part nevertheless overwhelmingly using a method of third-party payment—it is very bureaucratic. The absence of family doctors leads to duplication of effort (and expense), overinvestigation, lack of coordination in care, unnecessary and often harmful polypharmacy, and so forth.

The authors of the article are from the Commonwealth Fund, whose mission (beware of organizations bearing mission statements) is:

> to promote a high-performing health care system that achieves better access, improved quality, and greater efficiency, particularly for

society's most vulnerable, including low-income people, the uninsured,
minority Americans, young children, and elderly adults.

There is much that is worthy in this mission. Who, after all, would
be in favor of a low-performing health-care system or one with worse
access, lower quality and decreased efficiency? But intending good is
easy while doing good is difficult.

The value of the article was for me largely vitiated by a table based
upon a survey of health-care systems, ranking them in order of merit.
The countries surveyed were Australia, Canada, France, Germany, the
Netherlands, New Zealand, Norway, Sweden, Switzerland, the United
Kingdom and the United States. On most measures—overall ranking,
care process, access, administrative efficiency, equity and health-care
outcomes—the United States comes last or near to last, and the United
Kingdom comes first.

A glance at this table, however, ought to make people laugh. The
United Kingdom is first in overall ranking, first in care process and in
equity, third in access and in administrative efficiency, but next to last
(only the United States is worse) in health-care outcomes. In other
words, the United Kingdom equitably and efficiently administers very
nearly the worst health-care outcomes of those measured.

It surely requires a bureaucrat's-eye view of the matter to rank this
system first overall. From the no-doubt simplistic, naive and shallow
view of the average citizen, who does not understand that administrative process is vastly more important than outcome, the whole purpose
of a health-care system is to produce the best *outcomes* possible. This is
clearly not the more sophisticated view of the Commonwealth Fund.

Let us just take the criterion of equity. Almost certainly, equity as
the Fund understands it means equality, for otherwise fairness is too
difficult to measure. Is it fair that someone who has voluntarily indulged
in habits harmful to his health should impose the costs of having done
so on others? Does fairness in allocation of public funds for health care
necessitate a measure of the degree to which an individual is the author
of his own downfall? That is a very complex business, which would
inevitably lead to endless dispute and litigation.[1] But if equity is taken

---

1 Is an alcoholic, for example, fully, partially or not at all responsible for the deleterious
  health consequences of his heavy drinking? There is evidence of a genetic
  predisposition to drinking heavily, but also much evidence that people can stop if

to be equality, a complete absence of heath care would be equitable, and excellent health care for half the population but none for the other half would be grossly inequitable—though except for dogs in the egalitarian manger this would be an advance on a system that provided care for nobody.

But even on the matter of equality in the British health-care system the Commonwealth Fund is mistaken. For forty years before the institution of the famous (or infamous) National Health Service, the health differential between the richest and poorest was constant—the rich, of course, being healthier than the poor. As soon as the NHS was instituted, the differential began to increase, very slowly at first, but rapidly once the funding of the service was greatly increased. Of course, the differential might not have been *caused* by the NHS, but at the very least it is impossible to say that the NHS decreased inequality, though such was its justification and underlying intention.

And what of access to health care? In theory, it is equal under the NHS, but theory is not practice.[2] Let me relate a little anecdote to illustrate this.

I was asked to prepare a report on a 72-year-old man. He told me how, a short time before, he had experienced a sudden painful and reddened swelling in the calf of his leg, symptoms that a first-year clinical medical student ought to recognize as being of dangerous import. The man, a shy, mild-mannered retired manual worker, went to his doctor, where the receptionist told him that the doctor was too busy to see him. He therefore went to a pharmacy to buy some painkillers. Fortunately, the pharmacist asked him why he needed them, and he described his symptoms. The pharmacist telephoned his doctor and told him that he had better see this man. Only then did the man receive proper investigation and treatment (which may have saved his life). The point is,

they wish. There is further evidence that the price of alcohol, set by the government, affects the level of drinking in a population: that the cheaper it is, the more heavily people will drink. And drinking, of course, is only one determinant of health. Is a footballer to be held responsible for his own broken leg if he would not have had it but for playing football? How far does equity require that we take these calculations?

2 There was an interesting item in the *British Medical Journal* for March 3, 2018. Hospital deaths in England and Wales between 1997 and 2017 fell considerably further than in Scotland during the same period. In Scotland, officials had concentrated on improving access to and equality in care; in England and Wales, on the quality of care.

however, that no middle-class educated person would have tolerated being sent away in these circumstances by the receptionist, nor, probably, would the receptionist even have tried to do so.

While access to health care *de jure* is equal, *de facto* it is far from being so. This is not entirely the system's fault, however. For example, recall that prisoners in Britain have better chances of survival in prison than outside, according to standardized mortality ratios. One of the reasons for this (though not the only one) is that prison is the only place in which they seek health care, though it is freely available to them outside prison, every person in Britain having a doctor available to him as of right.

Curiously also, I have never heard any Western European speak of Britain's health service with anything other than fear or disgust, despite the Commonwealth Fund's ranking it first. No one in Western Europe says, when ill, "If only I were in Britain!" Rather, if they are ill in Britain, they do everything to be repatriated if at all possible. They regard the prospect of being treated under the NHS with terror. And oddly enough, the Commonwealth Fund ranks France's health-care system as next to last overall, worst in administrative efficiency and next to last in equity. This is indeed curious, since everyone I have spoken to in France is satisfied with the health care in their country (which has a very good reputation elsewhere also), however dissatisfied they may be about everything else.

It seems, then, that the members of the Commonwealth Fund live in a looking-glass world, where things are a mirror image of reality. But this is not quite the case, for the fact remains that the U.S. health-care system is costly and often inefficient. ▣

September 14, 2017

I t goes without saying (almost) that we all want the best medical treatment for ourselves and our loved ones—with the unacknowledged corollary that we want less than the best for other people, assuming that there will always be a variation between the best, average and worst medical treatment. I leave it to moral philosophers to decide whether this desire on our part is morally beneficial, reprehensibly selfish or merely natural.[1]

But how is one to go about finding the best treatment? On what grounds is one to judge? Fortunately for both doctor and patient, people are often convinced that they are receiving treatment from the very best person in the field: and insofar as faith in treatment is an important determinant of its success, perhaps it is more important to *believe* that one is receiving the best treatment than actually to receive the best treatment. This could only be true, of course, where the difference between the best treatment and the rest was not very great.

A paper in this week's *Journal*, titled "Hospital-Readmission Risk— Isolating Hospital Effects from Patient Effects," attempts to sort the hospital sheep from the hospital goats. This is important not only in itself but also because the American government wants to provide monetary incentives (including withholding of funds) for hospitals to improve their performance.

---

1 I think, though I may be doing him an injustice, that Professor Peter Singer of
   Princeton would find this desire morally illegitimate.

It is not easy, however, to compare hospital performance because of confounding factors. Some hospitals, being in poorer areas, will have sicker patients, and patients with less social support once they leave hospital. It is a comparatively late discovery in medicine that like must be compared with like for any valid conclusion to be drawn from a comparison. This may be obvious to us now, but it was not always obvious, self-evidence being a time-dependent phenomenon.

The authors of this paper, which is purely statistical in nature, took the 6,910,341 discharges from hospital under Medicare for the year 2014–15 and divided them into two random samples. They took the first sample of 3,455,171 discharges and ranked the hospitals from which the patients had been discharged into quartiles according to their rates of patient readmission for the same condition within thirty days of first discharge. (Since there were 4,272 hospitals, each quartile should have had 1,068 hospitals in it, but for some unexplained reason there were 1,101, 1,009, 1,021 and 1,141 hospitals in the quartiles instead.)

The remaining 3,455,170 discharges were winnowed down to a study sample of 37,508 patients who had had two admissions for similar diagnoses between one and twelve months apart, at different hospitals in different performance quartiles. The researchers used these dual-admission patients to compare quartile pairs (1 vs. 2, 3 vs. 4, etc.) in rates of thirty-day readmissions after their initial admissions of the same patients. In this way, the study controlled for characteristics of patients that may affect outcomes, so that differences in readmission rates could be attributed to quality of care.

Comparing the hospital quartiles in pairs, the researchers found a statistically significant difference in thirty-day readmission rates only between the best and the worst quartile when the same patients had been admitted to hospitals in both quartiles. This difference was 2 percent: there was one additional readmission in the worst hospitals for every fifty readmissions in the best. The question then arises whether this statistically significant difference is significant in any other, more important sense. After all, doctors treat patients, not statistics, even if patients are increasingly made to think that in the eyes of their doctor they are statistics rather than people; and significance to patients means "Will I feel better?" or "Will I live longer?" It does not mean "Is there a slight but reproducible difference on an analog scale of some measure or other?"

According to the authors, "This result may reassure the public, policymakers, and health care professionals that the signal of quality from the hospital-wide readmission measure is valid and can be used as a means to benchmark performance." These words seem to me to be a little ambiguous. The reassurance that the public, policymakers and health-care professionals *may* draw from the results could be the reassurance they *ought* to draw, or the reassurance it is possible that they *will* draw, whether misguided or not. The same ambiguity attaches to the use of the word *can*: it might mean *ought*, or it might mean *are able.*

The authors seem to favor the stronger sense, for they continue (and end): "Moreover, there may be opportunities for worse-performing hospitals to improve their care and avert potentially preventable readmissions." This is a rather odd conclusion, unless it is independently shown that readmission rates are a good and sufficient surrogate measure for some more important measure (from the patients' point of view), such as death rates. Perhaps this has already been done, but the authors make no reference to it, and do not even appear to notice that it is necessary. In other words, their minds have become so bureaucratic (though they are all Doctors of Medicine) that they appear to believe that the object of hospital treatment is to prevent readmission rather than death. After all, it is possible that readmission is a manifestation of something other than poor initial treatment, though it could be that.

The authors do admit that they have not calculated whether the 2 percent difference in readmission rates allegedly caused by the difference in quality of care is of minor significance compared with other factors affecting readmission rates, such as hospital size. Of all the hospitals examined, 69.8 percent had between one and 199 beds (how many had a solitary bed? one wonders), but only 55.8 percent of the worst performers, as measured by readmission rates, were of that size. By contrast, 6.6 percent of all the hospitals had more than 500 beds, but 11.4 percent of the worst performers were of that size.

There are also regional variations: while 38.7 percent of the hospitals were in the South, for example, 42.4 percent of the worst performers were in that region, and only 35.5 percent of the best.

Does this mean that a 77.5-year-old person in the South should take himself off to a hospital with fewer than 200 beds in the West or the Midwest, where the proportion of hospitals in the best quartile is higher? On the reasonable assumption that he is quite ill and frail, this might prove rather difficult. There are natural monopolies, or at least duopolies, in many places, so in fact the patient is hardly in a position to worry about whether the hospital to which he goes is in the best or the worst quartile with respect to readmission, which in any case is of relatively minor concern.

There are other problems with this way of assessing the performance of hospitals, of course. All the patients fell into one of five categories: surgical and gynecological, cardiovascular, cardiorespiratory, neurological, and "medical reasons" (a somewhat mysterious category, as one would hope that most admissions to hospital were for medical reasons). On the assumption that the patients fell more or less equally into these categories, an exceptionally bad performance in one of them could easily account for a difference of 2 percent in overall performance. The performance in the other four categories could be average or even above average. In the hospital in which I worked, the gastroenterologists were exceptionally good, but I wouldn't have sent a dog to the dermatologists.

The authors would no doubt reply that the purpose of their measure is not to inform individual patients about the quality of the hospital to which they should go if they want the best treatment, but rather as a signal, as they call it, to the administrators of the hospital system as a whole. A rising tide of quality is more important than the search for the very best hospital, since not everyone can be treated in the very best hospital, but an overall improvement in performance will benefit everyone, even those constrained to go to the worst hospital. This, it seems to me, is correct, though whether bureaucratic tinkering at the edges is what produces overall improvement is perhaps doubtful. After all, the use of anesthetics in surgery spread very rapidly without the intervention of hospital administrators, except to acquire the necessary chemicals. On the other hand, most medical progress these days is incremental rather than dramatic, not by giant leap but by small steps. Implementation of such steps may not be self-evidently desirable, as the use of anesthetics was.[2] Whether this paper represents even a small step—well, it is difficult to say. Further research is needed. ◙

---

2 It is a bit of a myth that anesthesia in childbirth was at first opposed because it went against biblical teaching that women should give birth in pain and suffering. The myth was assiduously spread by the self-promoting discoverer of chloroform, Sir James Young Simpson.

September 21, 2017

My most vivid memories of medical journals go back more than a third of a century, when I first read papers in the *Lancet* proposing, and then proving, that peptic ulceration was mainly an infectious disease. I was deeply skeptical at first, partly because it went against everything I had been taught and partly because my father had suffered from ulcers for decades and had tried various diets, pills and operations to relieve his suffering. The idea that he had experienced decades of severe pain that might have been ended by a simple course of drugs already in existence was hard to believe. But it was so.

Some years later I worked in a hospital in which one of the two leading cardiologists thought that coronary artery disease was also infectious. Perhaps he was after a Nobel Prize. If I remember rightly, *Chlamydia* was the organism that he most favored as a candidate. He also argued that the rise and fall in incidence of coronary artery disease was more characteristic of an infectious cause than any other. I did not dismiss his arguments out of hand as I might have done before peptic ulceration proved to be infectious.

In this week's *Journal*, there is an interesting trial that put me in mind of his theory in a Proustian way. The authors of the trial wanted to see whether a drug (a monoclonal antibody) that was designed to reduce inflammation in arteries would improve the prognosis of those who had already had a heart attack and who were therefore liable to have another, or a stroke. Inflammation has indeed been found to accompany coronary thrombosis, though whether as a cause or a consequence the authors do not state.

They enrolled 10,061 patients who had had heart attacks but no other obvious causes of inflammation, and divided them into four groups, one receiving a placebo and the others receiving varying doses of the treatment under trial, which was called canakinumab, by injection every three months. The researchers followed the patients for up to four years and found that both the biological marker of inflammation (a substance in the blood called C-reactive protein) and incidents such as heart attack or stroke, whether fatal or not, declined in frequency.

So far, so good: the treatment worked, then. But of course there is more to assessment of the value of a treatment than showing that it worked to a statistically significant extent. It has also to be shown that it worked to a clinically significant extent, which is a more important but not easily definable measure. Nor is that sufficient. It is possible to prolong a life while making it unbearable; it is also possible to save a life from one disease only to extinguish it by another. In practice, therefore, judgment is always necessary, and as Hippocrates informed us quite a long time ago, it is fallible.

The authors of the trial inform us that at the dose of canakinumab they found to be optimum (between the highest and lowest that they administered), there was a reduction of 0.64 events (stroke or heart attack) per 100 person-years. On the assumption that the patients on whom they tried the treatment had a life expectancy of ten years, for every 160 persons treated for a period of ten years, one of them would be spared a heart attack or stroke that he would otherwise have had. At the moment, there is no way of knowing which of those 160 patients will actually benefit from the drug.

What's more, the overall death rate in the treated and untreated groups was approximately the same; at least it was not different in the statistically significant sense, though it was slightly lower in the treated group. It might be that the difference in death rate was really attributable to the canakinumab, because statistical insignificance does not disprove clinical significance any more than statistical significance proves it. In any case, the difference was small.

The reason why there was no statistically significant improvement in the survival of the treated groups was that the treatment probably caused immunosuppression, leading to fatal infections. In other words, the treatment might have saved the patients from death by heart attack or stroke only to kill them by infectious disease.

There were a couple of passages, deeply buried in the paper where most busy doctors might not notice them, that caused me a moment's pause. In the section subtitled "Statistical Analysis," we read:

> The trial was designed to accrue a total of 1400 primary end-point events [heart attacks and strokes] across all the groups....The investigators initially sought to enroll 17,200 patients in order to accrue 1400 events over a period of 5 years. In December 2013, at the request of the sponsor, the sample size was reduced to 10,000 patients. The planned follow-up was extended by 1 year to maintain the targeted number of events.

The sponsor of the trial was Novartis, the manufacturer of the drug; and while the admission that there had been a change in its protocol suggests that there was nothing sinister in its request to lower the number of patients (otherwise, why even mention it?), the reasons for the change might have been worth a mention, in a time when the commercial corruption of intellectual and scientific integrity is so widely suspected.

The second passage that caught my attention was this:

> Six confirmed cases of tuberculosis occurred during the trial, with similar rates in the pooled canakinumab group and the placebo group; five cases occurred in India and one in Taiwan.

This is the first we hear of the trial's geographical location. Could it be that the majority of the patients in it were Indian? Drug companies have been accused in the past of using vulnerable populations for their trials, as it is cheaper, and there is less of a fuss when things go wrong, as they sometimes do. Small inducements to participate may be attractive to poor people. The dangers of litigation are lower, settlements are cheaper, and the ability to brush things under the carpet is greater. I do not say that any such considerations were important in the present trial, and I am not even absolutely sure that it would be morally wrong if they were. But still I was slightly taken aback.

To be fair, the trial was not expected to yield immediately applicable clinical results. It was what is called a *proof-of-concept* trial, an attempt to show that the theory on which it was based is not totally untenable. And this the trial did. It increased the likelihood that inflammation is causatively related to coronary artery disease. A judicious editorial accompanying the paper highlights the importance and the limits of the findings. It ends by saying:

> [This trial] has helped move the inflammatory hypothesis of coronary artery disease forward scientifically. However, the modest absolute clinical benefit of canakinumab cannot justify its routine use in patients with previous myocardial infarction [heart attack] until we understand more about the efficacy and safety trade-offs and unless a price restructuring and formal cost-effectiveness evaluation supports it.

⌣

Another article draws attention to the problems of tuberculosis elimination in the United States. In 1953, there were 52.5 cases per 100,000 of the population, and in 2016 only 2.9 cases per 100,000. This is a great success, of course, and all the more so since the rate had already declined dramatically by 1953.

But it is always possible, with a little determination, to derive bad news from good. A graph in the article shows that in 1993, foreign-born persons in the United States had a rate of tuberculosis five times that of native-born people. In 2016, the foreign-born had a rate of tuberculosis fourteen times that of the native-born. In the intervening quarter century, then, inequality had increased considerably in this respect. The *absolute* rate of tuberculosis among the foreign-born was halved during the same period, but this would be no cause for rejoicing among strict egalitarians, who prize equality as an end in itself. For them, everything can get better even as everything gets worse; and, conversely, everything can get worse while everything gets better. If equality is what you want, things were substantially better in 1993 than in 2016, when rates of tuberculosis were substantially higher for both native and foreign-born, but at least they were closer together. ▣

September 28, 2017

By strange coincidence, I happen to have read a strong implied criticism of one of the authors of the first research paper in this week's *Journal*, titled "Effects of Anacetrapib in Patients with Atherosclerotic Vascular Disease." The man criticized was Professor Rory Collins, director of the Clinical Trial Service Unit of Oxford University. The implicit criticism was that Collins and his unit were in the pocket of the Merck pharmaceutical company.

The author of the book *Too Many Pills* notes that "checking the outcomes in tens of thousands of participants in…clinical trials is a formidable task." It is also expensive. Concerning a trial of cholesterol-lowering drugs, he writes:

> How costly is not known, as drug company support…has never been declared—though [the] parent organisation, the Oxford University Clinical Trial Service Unit, has received £268 million over the past twenty years, £218 million contributed by just one company, Merck.[1]

As a result of his researches, Professor Collins went on to advocate the prescription of cholesterol-lowering drugs for an additional five million people in Britain alone, and in effect for scores of millions worldwide. By happy coincidence, the most commonly used drug to lower cholesterol was manufactured by Merck.

---

1 James Le Fanu, *Too Many Pills: How Too Much Medicine Is Endangering Our Health and What We Can Do about It* (London: Little, Brown, 2018), p. 110.

175

The trial discussed in the *NEJM* article was of a substance called anacetrapib, made by Merck. The company paid some of the expenses of the trial. In addition, we read, "Merck provided comments on the draft manuscript but otherwise had no role in the preparation of the manuscript or in the decision to submit for publication." None of this is proof of wrongdoing by anyone, but I have to admit that when I read the summary of the conclusions to this trial, a certain suspicion overtook me. The summary, or abstract, read as follows:

> Among patients with atherosclerotic vascular disease who were receiving intensive statin therapy, the use of anacetrapib resulted in a lower incidence of major coronary events than the use of placebo.

This is not a lie, but it is considerably less than the whole truth; and for the many busy doctors who read only the abstracts of papers, this creates a distinctly misleading impression. One is tempted to add that it is designed to do so.

There is no question about the admirable feat of organization that this paper reports. Unfortunately, feats of organization do not necessarily equate with scientific advance.

The authors arranged for hospitals around the world to conduct a double-blind trial of anacetrapib in 30,449 patients with proven atherosclerotic vascular disease who were also receiving statin therapy. (In essence, they aimed for a large number of patients because they knew in advance, or expected, the effect of the drug under investigation to be small. No one needed a trial of 30,000 patients to know whether or not penicillin worked.) Half of the patients received anacetrapib in a dose of 100 milligrams once daily, and the other half a placebo. The drug was designed to (and actually did) produce an increase in high-density lipoprotein cholesterol along with a reduction in low-density lipoprotein cholesterol. A high concentration of the former along with a low concentration of the latter is associated with a relatively low frequency of heart attacks; indeed, this association is believed by many to be causative. Hence, bringing such concentrations about might result in a reduction of heart attacks.

After four years, 1,640 of the 15,225 patients who had taken anacetrapib and 1,803 of the 15,224 patients who had taken placebo had suffered a major coronary "event" such as a heart attack or the need for revascularization by stent or coronary artery bypass graft. This means that out of 15,225 people taking a pill every day for a period of four years, 163 of them will avoid a heart attack or other major coronary "event" that they would otherwise have had.

The difference was statistically significant, but was it significant in any other way? The overall death rate, from both cardiac and non-cardiac causes, was the same in both groups: there were over 1,100 deaths in each. Admittedly, there was a tendency for the advantage of taking the drug to increase with time, so that if the trial had gone on for longer it might have produced better results. Even so, the results were hardly impressive; and it has to be remembered also that adherence to treatment is considerably greater during participation in trials than it is in "real life" situations, when a prescription becomes part of normal treatment.

If a patient were to ask, on the basis of this trial, whether or not he should take anacetrapib, what should the doctor tell him? The doctor could say that if he takes it for four years it will reduce his chances of a heart attack or need for revascularization, though not of dying, by 9 percent (one in eleven); or he could tell the patient that it will reduce his chances of a heart attack or need for revascularization by about 1 percent. Both are true, but I suspect that the former is more likely to induce someone to take the drug. How the doctor puts it will in part depend upon whether or not he wants his patient to take the drug. I confess that as I read the paper, wondering whether it might reveal a major advance in therapeutics, I could not help but think of lines from "The Walrus and the Carpenter" with regard to the sand on the beach.

> "If seven maids with seven mops swept it for half a year,
> Do you suppose," the Walrus said, "that they could get it clear?"
> "I doubt it," said the Carpenter, and shed a bitter tear.

By the way, there was no mention in the paper of the cost of anacetrapib, nor any mention of a trial against some other drug known or believed to reduce the occurrence of major cardiac events. The drug company would not have wanted that.

∽

Doctors more than most like to believe that they act rationally, especially on behalf of their patients. Often they do things that stand to reason, and that they therefore take for granted should be done. Swabbing the skin with an antibacterial prior to taking blood by needle and syringe is one such practice. I remember reading with horror that this practice serves no useful purpose whatever, and until the end of my career I felt uncomfortable about not swabbing the skin when taking blood.

Another thing that stands to reason is the provision of supplemental oxygen to people when they are suspected of having had a heart attack. After all, an insufficiency of oxygen is what causes the damage to the heart muscle in heart attacks, and so it makes sense that people suspected of having had one should be given oxygen to breathe. This has been believed for more than a hundred years. Oxygen supplementation has been standard treatment and is still recommended in treatment guidelines.

A paper from Sweden in this week's *Journal* undermines this venerable tradition. The authors divided patients suspected of heart attack and not suffering from a measurable deficiency of oxygen into two groups: in one, the patients were given supplemental oxygen for up to twelve hours; the others breathed normal air. The patients were followed up for a year to see if there was any difference in death rate or recurrence of heart attack.

The trial was a large one, with over 3,300 patients in each group. There was no difference between the groups either in death from any cause at 30 days or at 365 days after the suspected heart attack, or in rehospitalization for further heart attack at 30 or 365 days after the suspected heart attack. In the two groups, 5 percent and 5.1 percent of the patients, respectively, died within the first year, a difference much too small to be considered significant.

True, the trial was not double-blind or placebo-controlled: ordinary compressed air was not available to give to the patients by mask, nor could they be given a mask without such compressed air because they might have suffered from carbon dioxide retention if they had been. Nevertheless, the results seem definitive, insofar as any results in medical research can be. The trial demonstrated that the age-old practice served no useful purpose.

Or perhaps that is too sweeping a conclusion. I must admit that, even after reading this paper, I would rather like to have an oxygen mask if I were to have a heart attack. It would be like my teddy bear when I was young, the teddy bear for which I still feel an affection two-thirds of a century later. ◙

October 5, 2017

When my love swears that she is made of truth,
I do believe her though I know she lies,
That she might think me some untutored youth,
Unlearnèd in the world's false subtleties.
    —William Shakespeare, Sonnet 138

If asked to name the greatest medical advances of the second half of the twentieth century, few people, I imagine, would include the development and ever-greater utilization of the controlled trial for the assessment of the value of drugs and medical procedures. Nevertheless, this constitutes one of the most important changes ever to have occurred in the history of medicine. Until then, the evidence on which doctors based their treatment was either their own raw experience ("I have found oxygen bubbled through brandy to be helpful in pneumonia," a real example), or on the mere authority of others, itself based upon dubious claims. Surgery was rather better grounded than internal medicine, though its history was scattered with resort to unnecessary or hazardous operations, either for nonexistent conditions such as floating kidney, or for conditions that they did not cure.[1]

Another great change that came over medicine, especially in the last quarter of the century, was that doctors began to treat people not just for diseases they had, but for those they were at risk of developing in the future. Medicine became less curative and more preventive.

---

[1] The eminent surgeon Sir Arbuthnot Lane (1856–1943) was a great eviscerator to clean the "system" of toxins produced by the large bowel that supposedly caused all manner of problems—especially in those who could pay for the operations.

Immunization prevented diseases that were regarded as inevitable even during my own childhood, a normal part of growing up. By means of prevention, smallpox was eliminated, and the idea of prevention spread gradually to noninfectious diseases. High blood pressure being a causative factor in both heart attack and stroke, two of the great killers in advanced societies, it was thought that reduction of blood pressure in the susceptible population would reduce the incidence of both. To prove this, however, it was necessary to conduct trials on a large scale; and the smaller the anticipated benefit, the larger the trial had to be. You couldn't prove that taking blood pressure–lowering drugs was beneficial to those with only moderately elevated blood pressure by comparing a few patients who took such drugs with a few who did not.

But, as two *NEJM* articles this week inform the reader, the correct interpretation of trials is far from a straightforward matter. Indeed, such trials now rely on so great a statistical sophistication that the vast majority of doctors do not understand the basis on which they recommend treatments. They themselves are subject to a new kind of authority. It is frequently the case that reanalysis of trial results using different statistical methods produces different conclusions.

An article titled "Per-Protocol Analyses of Pragmatic Trials" is not such as to make the heart race with excitement, perhaps, and for me, a statistical illiterate, it was not an easy read—but certainly a worthwhile one. It made me consider things I had not really considered before, though I ought to have done so.

The results of most trials are analyzed on what is called an *intention-to-treat* basis: a group of patients is allocated to a treatment, and the result is expressed as a proportion of the whole group, irrespective of whether all members of the group actually took the treatment. For example, if 100 people with condition X are given treatment Y, which 20 of them for whatever reason do not take, or at least not for the whole length of the trial, and three-quarters of the remaining 80 are cured by it, the cure rate for the treatment is said to be 60 percent. A doctor relying on this conclusion, asked by a patient how effective his proposed treatment is, will say that it cures 60 percent of patients.

Using a *per-protocol* analysis of the results, however, the doctor would say that the treatment was curative in 75 percent of cases. The difference is important, because it might affect the patient's decision to take the treatment or not. While the per-protocol analysis might appear to be a more accurate measure of the treatment's effectiveness, we also need to know the reasons why 20 percent of patients in the trial dropped out. Perhaps it was because of intolerable side effects, but perhaps it was because they simply couldn't be bothered to continue. The difference between these two explanations is very important.

There are situations in which a per-protocol analysis is the more appropriate. The paper gives the example of a woman asking a doctor how effect is a certain method of contraception. No method of contraception works if it is not used properly, but clearly the woman who asks the question at least *intends* to use it properly. In this case, therefore, the doctor should reply using a per-protocol analysis, based on the numbers of those who adhered to the treatment.

But a raw per-protocol analysis of trial results is not the answer to all treatment dilemmas. The authors give the example of a trial of statins. Certain patients drop out of trials because of severe muscle pain or even rhabdomyolysis (a kind of dissolution of the muscles). Expecting them to complete the trial would be unreasonable and unethical, and omitting them from the analysis would be misleading. (I have seen deaths, possibly caused by the treatment, excluded from the analysis of results.)

A per-protocol analysis is particularly appropriate where the treatment is a simple procedure rather than a long-term consumption of drugs. The authors criticize an intention-to-treat analysis of the results of colonoscopy screening for colon cancer in Norway, because it underestimated the protective effect by including all those who were offered colonoscopy but refused it (about 30 percent). Clearly, no screening procedure can work for those who do not undergo it, and their choice has no bearing on its effectiveness per se.

But here the authors seem to have missed something. Whether the results of a screening procedure should be analyzed by per-protocol or intention-to-treat methods might depend on who is asking the question. The proper answer for an individual may be different from the answer most useful to a public health man who wants to know whether screening the whole population is a good idea. But it is even more complicated than this, for the proportion of people who refuse screening may be (probably is) dependent on the expected benefit to themselves.

Intention-to-treat analyses, by driving down the benefits to be expected from screening, may therefore turn into self-fulfilling prophecies of the ineffectiveness of screening. Of course, harms can be underestimated as well as benefits. The price of accuracy is eternal vigilance.

I thought that I (a complete amateur in these matters) spotted a mistake in the article's reasoning at one point. The authors referred to a trial in which the risk of death in those who adhered to a placebo was a statistically significant 10 percent lower than in those who stopped taking it. This is a very intriguing result. In order to conclude anything from it, of course, it is necessary to know that the only difference between those who did and did not adhere to treatment was in their adherence or failure to adhere. When the results were reanalyzed using new statistical methods, however, the difference between the adherers and nonadherers reduced to 2.5 percent. According to the authors, "the validity of these methods is easily verifiable in the reanalysis because we expect that the outcome should not be affected by adherence to placebo." If I am not mistaken, what this means is: decide the result, then choose the method. Since we know that adherence or nonadherence to placebo can have no real effect, therefore a statistical method that yields this result must be the correct one.

I have not exhausted the questions this interesting paper raises, nor those prompted by a sister paper, "Challenges in the Design and Interpretation of Noninferiority Trials."[2] Doing so would take a whole book, which I have neither the ability nor the energy to write. But in fact, no statistical analysis will answer all the questions that we have. Old Hippocrates was right after all: time is short, the art is long, the occasion fleeting and judgment difficult. ▪

---

2 These are trials in which it is attempted to show that a new treatment is not inferior to an old treatment that is already known to work. The new treatment, though not superior in effectiveness, may yet be safer or more convenient for the patient, and therefore, in effect, superior.

October 12, 2017

Modern intellectuals are divided into two camps: those (the majority) who think that there is no essential difference between man
and the rest of the living world, and for whom man is nothing but a
glorified insect or bacterium; and those (the minority) who think that
man's level of self-consciousness introduces something entirely new into
the universe—as far as we know. I belong to the minority.[1]

Among the differences between man and the animals is that man
is capable of contemplating his own total extinction, and even, of late,
enjoying that contemplation. It will occur by asteroid, by nuclear war
or by the emergence of a new infectious agent, most likely a virus. The
epidemic of Ebola virus disease in West and Central Africa raised the
specter of a new Black Death—sometimes with a not entirely unplea-
surable frisson among commentators.

This week's *Journal* has several articles about this fell disease, which
has nothing romantic about it at all. On the contrary, it is notably horrible and terrifying. As a way to die, Ebola is among the worst.

---

1 The majority view can crop up at odd times and in odd contexts. When I wrote
  this, I was in France and had bought the paper of bourgeois left-wing intellectuals,
  Libération (May 24, 2018). In it was an article about a new exhibition on the latest
  research concerning Neanderthal man. Here is a thought prominently and one
  supposes proudly displayed to attract readers: "Anthropophagy has long been the
  dividing line between the 'savage' and the 'civilised'. But, seeing images of the way
  animals are put to death in abattoirs, does a line still exist between carnivores and
  cannibals…?" Thus eating the flesh of animals and humans is equated.

The first article concerns the persistence of fractions (at least) of the Ebola virus in the semen of men who have recovered from the disease. There is nothing very reassuring in the findings. The authors tested the semen of 210 men in Sierra Leone who had recovered from the disease, which has a death rate that varies between 23 and 70 percent. At three months after recovery, all the men tested were positive for Ebola RNA in their semen; at 4 to 6 months, 62 percent of men tested were positive; at 7 to 9 months, 25 percent were positive; at 10 to 12 months, 15 percent were positive; at 13 to 15 months, 11 percent were positive; and at 16 to 18 months, 4 percent were positive. Admittedly, the numbers in each of the categories were small, and it cannot be known how representative they were of their respective groups, but two things about these results cause unease. The first is that Ebola is known to be transmissible by sexual intercourse; and second, the current recommendation for the period in which survivors of the disease should take precautions against sexual transmission is three months.

There are a couple of caveats, however. The first is that it is not known how often, or in what proportion of cases, the route of transmission is sexual. The second is that it is not known whether or how far the presence of Ebola RNA in the semen means that the person is infectious to others.

So terrifying and catastrophic is the disease, however, that these results might sow panic in countries in which the disease is now endemic. The fear of another epidemic is understandably great; and an accompanying article points out that survivors of the disease have already been discriminated against, evicted from their homes, dismissed from their jobs, quarantined and, in Sierra Leone, even imprisoned. If the only outcomes of Ebola virus disease are death or social ostracism, people with the disease, or their relatives, will not disclose its presence, and the reticence not only hampers public health measures to control the disease, but increases the death rate insofar as treatment can reduce it. Word of the research findings on the persistence of the virus in the semen of convalescents is bound to reach the affected countries sooner or later, and a simplistic interpretation (survivors remain dangerous for a long time) is likely to predominate. It is not only in the modern Western world that the precautionary principle is taken in earnest.

Serious and necessary scientific work can thus have a deleterious effect, at least for a time. The truth will not necessarily set you free.

Another paper reports the results of controlled trials of two vaccines against Ebola virus. Both successfully evoked an immune response that endured for at least twelve months. This is encouraging, but not definitive; what needs to be known is whether the vaccines in practice actually protect against contraction of the disease. It is not an immune response per se that is desired.

The difficulty of conducting definitive trials in the middle of an epidemic such as that of Ebola are the subject of another article. This applies to putatively therapeutic agents as well as to vaccines. In the midst of a catastrophic and terrifying epidemic, would it be ethically permissible to withhold possibly life-saving agents from anyone? And even if it were ethical, would anyone agree in these circumstances to enter a trial involving the use of placebo?

In theory, it would be possible to conduct trials using past outcomes of the disease—past death rates—as a control. But this is far more difficult than might at first appear, because those death rates themselves vary considerably, in part because it has been found that ordinary medical supportive methods, where available, such as intravenous infusion, reduce the death rate. Treatment of concomitant malaria, very common in the areas in which Ebola spreads, affects the death rates, and even the combination of drugs used to treat malaria does so. In other words, trials are conducted against a moving target.

Although the article about the difficulties of conducting trials in the midst of an epidemic is titled "We Can Do Better" (would any article with the title "We Have Done the Best We Can" be published?), I find the work already done impressive. After all, people have risked their lives that it might be done.

There is a dog that did not bark in the nighttime in a paper titled "Romosozumab or Alendronate for Fracture Prevention in Women with Osteoporosis." This was a trial of two drugs, which showed that women at high risk of fracture who took romosozumab had a substantially lower rate of fracture than those who took alendronate. The trial assumed that alendronate, a now-standard treatment, was itself beneficial in the prevention of fractures.[2] In a follow-up of two years, romosozumab prevented 5.7 percent of women from suffering a vertebral fracture, and 3.3 percent of them from having any fracture at all. The percentage of women suffering from the most dangerous fracture of all in such a susceptible population, that of the hip, was reduced from 3.2 percent to 2.0 percent.

These are excellent results—provided, of course, that they are not obtained at the cost of adverse effects that outweigh the good. Here, it seems to me, matters become more equivocal, and even sinister. I quote:

> An imbalance in adjudicated serious cardiovascular adverse events was observed...with 50 patients (2.5%) in the romosozumab group and 38 (1.9%) in the alendronate group reporting these events....A total of 16 patients (0.8%) in the romosozumab group and 6 (0.3%) in the alendronate group reported cardiac ischemic events and 16 patients (0.8%) in the romosozumab group and 7 (0.3%) in the alendronate group reported cerebrovascular events....

These differences are not statistically significant, which however does not necessarily mean that they are not real. Interestingly (at least to me), the death rate in the romosozumab group was over 40 percent higher than in the alendronate group, a fact which was not even mentioned in the paper and which, if real, would mean an extra four deaths in 1,000 people taking romosozumab by comparison with those taking alendronate.

It is true that this difference in death rates might not be real; and the authors refrain from testing whether it is statistically significant. But it is also true that they believe the difference—or *imbalance*, as they delicately call it - in cardiovascular events, meaning strokes and heart attacks, is a real one. Why such coyness about death?

Could it possibly have anything to do with the fact that the trial was funded by the companies that made romosozumab, that two of the three writers of the paper were employees of those companies, that the paper was written "with medical-writing assistance funded by" the companies,

---

2 For a criticism of the routine use of alendronate, see Le Fanu, *Too Many Pills*, pp. 217–23.

and that the "trial investigators signed agreements with the sponsors relating to data confidentiality"?

Perish the thought.

While on the subject of euphemism, I wonder why the authors of the paper on the persistence of Ebola RNA in the semen felt it necessary to say that their subjects were *financially compensated* rather than *paid*. We laugh at the Victorians, but not at ourselves. ▣

October 19, 2017

One of the complaints of doctors worldwide is of the increasing bureaucratization of their profession. They study for years and end up spending half their time filling forms of no immediate benefit to their patients. It is not for this that they chose the profession, and they quickly become disillusioned and even cynical because of it. They often feel, into the bargain, that they are being controlled by people inferior to themselves both morally and intellectually. And this is so regardless of how health care is arranged, what system is in place, and the varying opinions or outlook of doctors on other subjects.

Members of other professions also complain of increasing bureaucracy, so perhaps there must be something in the zeitgeist propitious to it. But in the case of medicine there are three factors that make it almost inevitable. First, there is the ever-increasing technological sophistication and therefore expense of medicine. Second, there is the ever-greater intrusion of information technology into our world; and if information can be gathered, it will be gathered. Third, there is the ever-decreasing proportion of the population that can pay directly for its medical care. Intermediaries such as insurance companies and governments feel obliged to obtain the best value for money they can. But what is the best value for money and how is it to be measured? If different desiderata are incommensurable, if even in principle there is no single unit of measurement to which they can all be reduced, the task is fundamentally impossible, even though it must be undertaken. Waste is probably easier to spot than value.

A paper in this week's *Journal* looks into whether any benefit would accrue from expanding the Hospital Readmissions Reduction Program in the United States. The HRRP currently imposes financial penalties on those hospitals with higher-than-average readmission rates for five specified causes of admission, and the authors set out to estimate the results of extending it to cover readmission rates for practically all causes. The penalty comes in the form of reductions in the reimbursement of hospitals for patients treated in them under Medicare and Medicaid. There is no positive financial reward for performing better than average.

Would a carrot work better than a stick? In Britain, a system of paying general practitioners (family doctors) if they achieve specified targets—such as a proportion of their patients in certain categories treated according to a protocol decided by the government—has fundamentally altered the nature of medical consultations, such that (generally unbeknown to patients) what the doctor does to them is not what *he* thinks best for them, but what the government has, in effect, bribed him to do. Mass prescription has been incentivized, often on the basis of marginal evidence, as has lying, for the information that is gathered is treated as if it must be true, and it is easy to falsify records. The scale of falsification is unknown, and perhaps for the moment it remains relatively small; but it is unwise to rely on moral capital to expect honesty when the furnishers of information are becoming more and more cynical or disillusioned.

Under the HRRP, which is part of the Affordable Care Act (whose very title assumes that it *will* result in what it is designed to produce), hospitals may receive up to 3 percent less money for treating five categories of in-patients on Medicare or Medicaid if their readmission rate is deemed higher than it should be. The categories are myocardial infarction (heart attack), pneumonia, heart failure, hip or knee replacements, and chronic obstructive airway disease.

In order for such a system to be fair, like has to be compared with like. Those hospitals with high proportions of Medicare and Medicaid patients, which the authors call *safety-net hospitals*, were likely to be in relatively impoverished areas, where prognoses are usually poorer than in rich areas independently of treatment received. Poor people, for example, now smoke more than rich—the high taxation on cigarettes notwithstanding—and of course smoking is one of the most important factors in a poor prognosis. Therefore, complex adjustments have to be made in adjudicating performance even on the simple measure of readmission rates. Furthermore, only hospitals with a certain level of activity within the categories are eligible (if that is the word) for penalties; otherwise the numbers would be too small for drawing proper conclusions from them.

The HRRP appears to have worked insofar as hospital readmission rates for the categories in which penalties apply have fallen, particularly in safety net hospitals. Perhaps this is not surprising, since those are the hospitals in which penalties are potentially most onerous. A causative relationship between financial penalties and falling readmission rates is assumed, because readmission rates declined more for targeted conditions than for others, though this is not itself decisive proof of such a relationship. And the five targeted categories, plucked from the air by medico-bureaucrats, cover only a small proportion of a hospital's activity. Why not include the total hospital readmission rate in the calculations for financial incentives? Would this not drive down readmission rates even further—indeed, much further?

Prima facie, hospital-wide readmission rates would be a better target than the rates in five selected categories, for two main reasons. First, if you select only certain conditions as the basis for imposing a financial penalty, a hospital could funnel resources disproportionately into treating those particular conditions, to the detriment of other types of patient. Second, because the numbers are much larger for hospital-wide readmissions, they can be a reliable measure within a shorter time, and therefore penalties can apply much sooner. Punishments are, of course, more effective the closer they are in time to the conduct that occasions them.

The authors of the article estimate what would happen if the HRRP were applied to practically all (93 percent) of acute admissions to hospital. To begin with, their data revealed a surprisingly small difference between safety-net hospitals and other hospitals in current readmission rates for all acute admissions: 15.8 percent against 15.2 percent. This suggests to me that differences in treatment are rather small, and that the primary determinant of medical care is the nature of the condition treated—which is as it should be. Nevertheless, a 0.6 percent difference among millions of hospital admissions means substantial absolute numbers of patients: 6,000 per million.

The authors come to the conclusion that if the program were extended to cover all, or nearly all, acute hospital admissions, there would be only a small increase in the number of hospitals that are penalized, though penalties for safety-net hospitals would rise substantially (from about $133,000 to $551,000).

What the authors do not consider is whether any of the bureaucratic activity involved in the program actually benefits patients. This was undoubtedly not the question that they set out to answer, but it is one that doctors and patients would like the answer to: for if the answer is no, all the complex calculations and adjustments in the world are of no interest or importance.

At first sight it might seem obvious that a lower readmission rate is beneficial, insofar as it implies better initial treatment. But at best it is only a proxy measure for that improvement, and it could even be a sign of deterioration in overall care. This is because the decision to readmit a patient is determined not only by his immediate medical state but also by his circumstances: his access to good primary care, for example, or his social isolation. A decline in the rate of readmissions might therefore be as much a sign of increased callousness or failure to take the overall situation of the patient into account, as an indication of improvement in care—all the more so when there is a financial incentive involved. The incentive could encourage callousness as much as good medical care; for when bureaucrats set a target, it is the target that is targeted, not the thing for which it is supposed to stand as proxy. Those who spend their day poring over statistics are rarely thinking of individual human suffering.

I am not saying that this *is* the case here: it might or might not be. But there is no sign of an awareness of the possibilities in the paper itself. By the way, death decreases the readmission rate most effectively. ◼

October 26, 2017

"A well regulated Militia, being necessary to the security of a free State, the right of the people to keep and bear Arms, shall not be infringed." Perhaps no single sentence, at least in relatively plain English, has ever aroused more interpretative controversy or confusion than the Second Amendment to the United States Constitution. Certainly none arouses more passion in the contemporary United States.

An editorial in the *Journal* meditates upon the mass shooting that happened in Las Vegas on October 1, which was then the latest and worst such outrage in American history, though destined not to be the last (and this would probably not be the last *NEJM* editorial on the subject, either). Whatever else people might suppose the Second Amendment to have meant in the minds of those who framed it, it could not possibly have meant the right of a man to spray a large number of people attending a music festival with automatic rifle fire from a quarter of a mile away, killing 59 and injuring 500.[1]

What do doctors have to say on the matter qua doctors, rather than merely as citizens? In my opinion, not very much. The editorial writers, knowing how passionate Americans are on the subject, manage to say very little that any reasonably intelligent person could not have worked out for himself. Pointing out that "our current political leadership [both Democrat and Republican] is apparently not willing to promote gun-violence prevention of any kind," they add, with startling bathos, "And

1 Anders Breivik in Norway killed more but injured fewer.

yet no one in America wants more mass shootings"—except, presumably, those very few who perpetrate them, some of whom, at least, seem intent on beating the record for the number of victims.

But what will prevent mass killings? The authors fall back partly on that old medical favorite, more research is needed: "One area for potential consensus is on the need for more research on how to reduce deaths from gun-related violence and how to prevent mass shootings." Earlier they suggested that tighter background checks on those applying for gun licenses "can keep war weapons out of the hands of those who are known to be mentally unstable." This might indeed be so, but the problem is that mentally unstable persons make up only a very small proportion of those who perpetrate such shootings, and in the case of the perpetrator of the latest outrage, "this 64-year-old man had no known political, racial, or religious agenda, and there was no history of known mental illness or criminal behavior."

There are things the editorial does not dare say, though I suspect that the authors (editors of the journal, not scholars of the subject) would have liked to say them. The Second Amendment was framed at a time when no one, not even the government, had weapons that could have done what was done in Las Vegas, and probably no one at the time even envisaged the possibility of such weapons. Moreover, the purpose of the right to bear arms was probably twofold, possibly threefold: the two most important purposes, given the preamble about a well-ordered militia being essential etc., were first to defend the country, and second to prevent a prepotent tyrannous central government or have means to overthrow it if it developed. The third purpose might have been for individual self-defense, but a society in which extremely potent weapons capable of killing people at a great distance were necessary for self-defense would be one so horrible that it would not be worth defending.

The United States is not protected from external enemies by the prevalence of gun ownership, but by its armed forces, the power of which the Second Amendment was intended to make unnecessary; and the disparity between the power of the government and that of armed citizens who might try to overthrow it by insurrection would be like hunting *Tyrannosaurus rex* with a pea-shooter. Into the bargain, the American government, along with all other modern democratic governments, is vastly more intrusive in the life of its citizenry than the colonial government ever was, for purely technical reasons. Recognition of this greater intrusiveness has induced individuals or small groups of *enragés* to try to live in autarky, as frontiersmen might have lived two centuries ago, but they are a tiny minority, mainly regarded as mad in the loose sense.

Finally, the Second Amendment was proposed at a time when it was not even certain who constituted *the people* whose right was not to be infringed (the United States then having a narrower franchise than did Great Britain). It is now completely obsolete, at least if its original intentions are what determines its present salience. But to suggest this would be almost like suggesting to a Moslem that God does not exist and Mohammed was not his prophet.

However, even if the Second Amendment were repealed on the grounds of obsolescence (a political impossibility), there would still be the question whether it would serve any purpose to do so, at least from the standpoint of preventing mass shootings. After all, automatic weapons are largely prohibited anyway, but it seems that people—that is to say, mass killers—experience little difficulty in obtaining them. As far as gun control in the United States is concerned, it resembles shutting the stable door after the horse has bolted. There are as many guns in private ownership as people in the country, although their ownership is not evenly spread. It is inconceivable that a person determined to be a mass killer would encounter very much difficulty in obtaining the wherewithal to achieve his ambition. No attempt at reducing the number of guns would be likely to have a substantial effect on the frequency of what are still rare events.

The feebleness of the editorial's conclusion is understandable: "Even in our dangerously polarized political system, there has to be a way for good people to come together on common ground and act." Why has there to be? Because one would like there to be? Because it is inscribed in human nature?

A small item, in the form of a letter, caught my attention for two reasons, one personal and one scientific. "The Success of Sinister Right-Handers in Baseball" was a reply to a letter published in the *Journal* in

1982 (thirty-five years ago!) that had drawn attention to the relative success of left-handers in professional baseball.

I am left-handed myself, and left-handers are less fully lateralized in cerebral function than right-handed people; in other words, the functions of the right and left hemispheres of the brain are less differentiated. The authors of the 1982 letter claimed that this gave left-handed players who both batted and threw left-handed an advantage over those who batted left-handed but threw right-handed, who in turn had a better performance record than those who both batted and threw right-handed.

The authors of the new letter, who surprisingly came from countries (the Netherlands, Germany, Britain) where baseball is not played, reanalyzed the original data provided in the first letter and came to a very different conclusion. They found that the advantage (in batting) was greatest for those who batted left-handed but threw right-handed, and that this advantage was greater than found in the previous research for all left-handed batters. The explanatory hypothesis of the authors is biomechanical rather than neurological. The arm with which people throw, especially if they practice, is generally stronger than the other arm. Therefore, the stronger right arm in left-handed batters who throw right-handed is held lower down the bat, and this gives them a longer lever with which to hit the ball.

My own lateralization is clearly incomplete. I write with my left hand and kick with my left leg, but if I want to throw something far I use my right arm. If I want to throw something a short distance but very accurately, however, I use my left arm. I hasten to add that my own career in sports was undistinguished, but biomechanics had nothing to do with it. I could never take sport seriously as a human endeavor.

There is also a more general lesson to take from this short item, an important and perhaps not entirely reassuring one. Reanalysis of data—in this case, relatively simple data—can produce a very different conclusion from the one originally drawn, and the reanalysis may not be done for many years. In the meantime, doctors have been acting upon the analysis that is later shown to be faulty. Then again, a reanalysis of the reanalysis may show it to be faulty as well.

What is truth, said jesting Pilate, and would not stay for an answer. ◾

November 2, 2017

The confusion between inequality and inequity is now chronic. They are not the same, for it is perfectly obvious that equity may result in inequality, and indeed might necessarily do so. An enforced equality would be inequitable, for it would take no account of individual effort or merit. On the other hand, inequality may result from inequity, and has often done so. Inequality is easy to measure; inequity is difficult to assess.

The confusion is once again clearly illustrated in an article in this week's *Journal*—if confusion can be said to be clear. The article is titled "A Renewed Focus on Maternal Health in the United States." It draws attention to the discomfiting and possibly scandalous fact that the maternal mortality rate (defined as the number of deaths occurring in 100,000 pregnant women or women who have given birth in the preceding 42 days) in the United States is now more than twice, and approaching three times, that in Canada. Furthermore, contrary to the trend in other developed countries, it has risen sharply of late. In 1995, it was 11 per 100,000, similar to Canada's rate today. In 2013 (the latest date cited in the article) it was 28 per 100,000.

Naturally there are inequalities within the United States between different sections of the population, but on almost every occasion they are referred to in the article as inequities. Whether inequalities are inequitable depends upon how they arise. Would anyone say that the gross overrepresentation of blacks in European football teams (which almost guarantees them the status of millionaire), by comparison with the number of blacks in the general population, is an inequity? An inequality of outcome between groups, whether for good or ill of the groups, does not in itself prove that an injustice has been committed.

How is it that the United States has so high a maternal mortality rate (for a developed country, that is), and moreover one that is rising? Part of the reason, the authors suggest, is a change in the way deaths are recorded. The authors state:

> Improvements in data collection (for example, the addition of a pregnancy question and checkbox on death certificates and *International Classification* of *Diseases* diagnostic codes) have increased detection of maternal deaths and may have led to overreporting in some cases.

It is a strange improvement in data collection that leads to inaccuracy, but let that pass. In addition, the authors do not address the question whether the same changes in data collection have occurred in other countries, so we are left guessing as to whether this change could or could not account for at least some of the divergence of the United States from the rest of the developed world.

The authors consider other factors that might account for the rising maternal mortality rate, chief among which are increasing obesity, high blood pressure and diabetes in young women, which themselves are strongly associated with poverty. Cardiovascular disease is now the most common cause of maternal death. Increasing rates of caesarean section (for whatever reason, good or bad) also increase maternal death rates. Again, the authors do not address the question whether these changes have occurred in other countries where similar increases in maternal mortality rates have not occurred.

They write: "As deeply troubling as the overall rise in maternal mortality are the inequities in maternal outcomes in the United States." According to one analysis of the statistics in twenty-seven states, the maternal mortality rate of black women is nearly three times that of white women (56.3 versus 20.3 per 100,000). Having referred to this data, the authors continue:

> The reasons for these disparities are poorly understood and undoubtedly complex; they include social determinants of health and biases

in care delivery. But such inequities signal that we can do far better for the most disadvantaged women.

Here disparities slide into inequities by means of "social determinants," though whether those social determinants are themselves inequitable is not asked, let alone proved.[1] Moreover, if inequality in outcome was what mattered, then equity in the sense meant in the article might be served by increasing the maternal mortality rate of white women, and by denying them prenatal care until it reached the levels that black women have. I take it that no one would suggest such a proceeding in the name of equity.

Does this mean that we must be like the three monkeys who hear, see and speak no evil in the face of these discomfiting statistics? That we are compelled to a Buddha-like calm? I do not think it means this in the slightest. The reason that the statistics are discomfiting is not that they indicate inequality or inequity, but because they indicate suffering (for behind every death there is a tragedy); and moreover it is suffering that might be alleviated or prevented altogether. It seems to me highly likely that many of the deaths might have been averted by proper medical care, and wherever such deaths can be averted, they ought (within the bounds of reason) to be averted—not in order to produce equality of outcome, but to reduce suffering. In this article, interestingly, there is not once a reference to unnecessary or avoidable suffering.

If it is suffering rather than inequality that is the target, does this mean that no special efforts should be made to see that black women get proper medical care? Again, not at all. As a general rule, it is easier and cheaper to improve the health of people starting at a low level than it is to improve the health of people who are already healthy. In the abstract, I am not a complete utilitarian: I think there are some deontological principles of morality. One does not kill every person the world would be better off without on the grounds of maximizing utility. But I doubt that anyone can altogether escape utilitarian calculations in trying to decide what to do; and if the enterprise of medicine as a whole has at

---

1 Thus what is poorly understood becomes a symptom of inequity. This is an illustration of the modern determination to find inequity in practically everything, as being the touchstone of moral philosophy.

least something to do with the reduction of as much suffering and the prolongation of as much life as possible, which I think it impossible to deny, it would make sense to direct extra effort toward black women, even if at least some of their suffering and premature death is the predictable consequence of their own choices.

⤺

The very next *NEJM* article suggests that considerations of equity, in the sense meant by the preceding authors, are in certain circumstances not ethically important. The article, "Dreams Deferred—The Public Health Consequences of Rescinding DACA," concerns the Deferred Action for Childhood Arrivals program, introduced by executive order during President Obama's first term of office.[2]

Under DACA, immigrants who were brought to the United States before the age of sixteen are immune from deportation and can receive work permits, provided that they are in school, have received a high school diploma, or have served in the military, and have no significant criminal record. I think these provisions are reasonable and humane, and would be deleterious only if the economy were a cake of fixed size, such that a job for a beneficiary of DACA implies one job less for a native-born American. The authors of the article report on the "mental health" benefits that DACA brings to its beneficiaries, such as a reduction in their levels of anxiety. (Of course, burglars would feel much less anxiety if there were no police.)

But DACA is also highly discriminatory, and rests on the assumption that such qualities as law-abidingness and attention to education are desirable and under voluntary control. Gone is the idea that equity requires an equal outcome for all, irrespective of conduct, and that all should be granted the same legal rights however they have behaved. The purpose of DACA, I presume, is to encourage good behavior and deter bad, and to encourage and reward effort. It is thus inequitable in the previous article's sense, but it is equitable in mine.[3] ◾

---

2 The authors do not consider the question whether such an arrangement—whether it be good or bad, but that touches upon a matter of importance to the American people—ought to be introduced by presidential fiat. It seems that one is in favor of authoritarianism if the authority does things that one approves of.

3 Provided that beneficiaries do not use it as an argument for family reunification.

November 9, 2017

I deally, changes in medical practice should proceed from evidence. This might seem so obvious as not to be worth saying, but for most of medical history, changes in practice were not the result of anything that we should nowadays recognize as evidence. Extraneous factors were more important, for example, the persuasiveness or charisma of the doctor proposing the change. Conviction carried weight.

Between 1996 and 2013, at least in California, an ever-growing proportion of the heart valves used in surgical replacement of defective valves were of biological origin rather than mechanical, increasing from 11.5 to 51.6 percent for the aortic valve, and from 16.8 to 53.7 percent for the mitral valve. Was this change justified by the superior results of valves of biological origin?

A paper in this week's *Journal* tries to answer this question. At first sight, it might seem easy to do so, but in fact it is very complex because there are so many variables to be taken into account. The question is important because, with an aging population, valvular disease (especially aortic) is becoming more prevalent, and patients are increasingly inquisitive about what is best for them. Mostly they want a nice simple answer.

The authors examined the results of aortic or mitral valve replacements in 142 hospitals in California from the beginning of 1996 to the end of 2013. They were mainly interested in what they called their "primary end point," which was "mortality." It is, indeed, quite an important end point—the end point of us all; though in some studies in the *Journal* it appears to be somewhat overlooked. The authors were induced to perform their study by the fact that previous studies of the same kind claimed that there were no differences in death rates between those given biological and those given mechanical replacement valves, but obviously they did not quite believe it. Those studies were too limited to have detected small but statistically significant differences in mortality. The authors of the present study also had secondary end points: rates of bleeding, stroke, perioperative mortality and reoperation. Because mechanical valves require lifelong treatment with anticoagulants, which biological valves do not, it is already known, and uncontroversial, that hemorrhage and stroke are more common with mechanical valves.

The numbers of people undergoing such operations might surprise you. There were 43,639 who underwent aortic valve replacement and 38,431 who underwent mitral valve replacement during the study period in those 142 hospitals. In the subsequent analysis of the results, however, the majority of these patients were excluded, either because they were not California residents (I cannot see the immediate relevance of this), or because they had had previous heart surgery, including previous heart valve surgery, or thoracic aorta surgery. The exclusions reduced the number of patients to only 9,942 in the case of aortic valve replacement and 15,503 in that of mitral valve replacement. Oddly enough, the authors make no mention of this high rate of exclusion in their discussion of the results, or the limitation it places on their usefulness or generalizability. It is one of the cardinal rules of valid comparison that like must be compared with like, so the results discussed here apply only to patients similar to those included in the study. Strictly speaking, this paper can help to inform decisions only with a minority of patients eligible for valve replacement surgery.[1]

The researchers divided their patients further into age groups, for it has been suggested that the long-term results of surgery differ according to age. The death rate for patients between 45 and 54 years

---

1 Trials have already established the value of such surgery. This is not the same, however, as saying that the surgery that is actually performed is beneficial. As the criteria for any treatment are loosened, so the results of trials establishing the value of that treatment become less and less applicable. Medical practice is a complex matter.

.

of age given biological aortic valves was higher than that of those given mechanical valves: 30.6 percent versus 26.4 percent.[2] This is statistically significant, and means that patients lived almost six months longer. The difference disappeared for patients over the age of 55.

The difference was considerably greater where mitral valves were concerned. Here, for patients from 44 to 49 years of age, the death rate for those given biological valves was nearly twice that of those given mechanical: 44.1 percent against 27.1 percent. Between the ages of 50 and 69, the difference was smaller, 50 percent against 45.3 percent, but still statistically significant, equating to more than 190 days of life per patient. Once patients were 70 or older, the difference disappeared.

Reoperation was more frequently required by those who had biological valves, but both hemorrhage and stroke were, as expected, more common among those given mechanical valves. Rather frustratingly, the paper version of the *Journal* omits to tell us just how common, though the figures can be found in the electronic version. It is not just the numbers of strokes that one needs, however, but their severity and density. What extra chance of a stroke, and how long endured in its consequences, is equal to six months of extra life? This question is probably not susceptible to a conclusive answer.

It seems to me probable, however, that the mechanical valves are superior at least for younger patients, which is in contradiction to the trend toward biological valves. But further research may produce a different result; and since this analysis covers a prolonged period, it is possible that the situation will evolve. The target—the best possible advice to patients—is a moving one, and surgeons will continue to be guided by their own experience and predilections as well as by papers such as this.

Every week, the *Journal* publishes photographs, both clinical and artistic, so to speak. The latter, taken by doctors, are usually lyrical in nature, illustrating the magnificence or beauties of nature. I surmise that the

2 The follow-up period varied greatly, of course, according to when the operations were performed in the time span from 1996 to 2013.

aspects of nature with which doctors habitually deal are ugly or upsetting, metaphorically red in tooth and claw, and therefore they take refuge in photographing its beauties in order to remind themselves that there is more to nature than pathology. This week there is a picture of the great migration of the wildebeest, I suspect (though the location is not mentioned) in the Serengeti in Kenya or Tanzania. This annual migration is a marvel to behold and restores one's faith in the beneficence of existence.

On the opposite page, however, is a clinical picture, or rather three clinical pictures, which are less aesthetically pleasing. They show a condition called compartment syndrome, which occurs when blood seeps into the space between muscles because of crush injury or prolonged pressure and immobility. This accumulation of blood interferes with blood supply to the muscles and nerves, and unless it is released, the muscles become gangrenous and the nerves in effect are killed.

The case illustrated in the photographs was that of a young man with compartment syndrome in his left forearm. He presented to hospital in Dublin with a swollen, painful left hand, and movement in his forearm was prevented by pain both on active and passive movement. His radial pulse—that felt at the wrist—was not palpable. He underwent emergency surgery to decompress the arm, and there were pictures of his arm when he arrived, and of the musculature in his forearm before and after operation, when circulation had been restored.

It was the few details of the case (apart from the pictures themselves) that drew my attention to it. Here was the cause of his compartment syndrome: "He had been lying on the ground for more than 13 hours after using illicit drugs." A second operation was performed 48 hours later to close the gaping open wound produced by the first with a split skin graft. "The patient did not participate in recommended hand therapy, and hand stiffness and paresthesia [pins and needles] persisted. He was subsequently lost to follow-up."

One can lead a patient to treatment, but one cannot make him take it. Although in this case the patient's lack of cooperation would irritate any doctor, nevertheless the patient's freedom to do the wrong thing and not to follow sound advice reassures me that we humans are not mere machines that invariably estimate what best to do according to a felicific calculus. ▣

November 16, 2017

Sport is generally regarded as a healthy and health-giving activity, especially in these days of expanding waistlines and metabolic syndrome. In my youth it was also regarded as character building, especially when it involved physical discomfort. There was nothing like scraping your knees on hard frozen ground to put virtuous iron in your soul.

I never really believed it, and though by no means incompetent at sport, I could not take it seriously enough to train or practice conscientiously. I did not observe that those who were very good at it, or trained hard, were of superior character to others. If anything, there seemed to me an inverse relationship between decency and sporting prowess. Sport gave license to bullies.

In the modern world, sport is an important aspect of the regime of bread and circuses. The excitement that people derive from sport is often proportional to the boredom of their lives and has an almost hysterical or simulated quality to it. Crowd behavior is frequently unattractive, and deaths in rioting occasioned by a match of some kind are far from unknown. Sport inflames nationalist passions of the crudest kind. Wasteful public expenditure on international sporting extravaganzas occurs repeatedly, leaving a legacy of debt and buildings of scarce utility but expensive upkeep. Competitive sport is also a gift to ideological or totalitarian regimes, which use sporting victory as a proof of philosophical superiority over their enemies.

Nor is this all. Sport is one of the most important causes of injury in the world. In one survey of adolescent participants in competitive sport, 65 percent were either injured, or had been injured in the past. What other activity would be permitted with so high a rate of causing harm to young people? There must be some very strong prejudice acting in favor of its continuation and encouragement in the face of so much harm done.

A paper from Canada in this week's *Journal* examines the question of sudden cardiac death in young people (defined as being from 12 to 45 years old) while indulging in sporting activities, competitive or noncompetitive. Previously, the incidence of sudden cardiac death during sporting activity was reported as 0.46 per 100,000 per year, about half the risk of being murdered in a country such as Britain or France. Could cardiac health screening of participants reduce the risk of such deaths?

The authors examined all the cases of cardiac arrest in people between 12 and 45 years of age that occurred outside of hospital in an area of Ontario with a population of 6.6 million inhabitants, of whom 3.09 million were in that age group. A cardiac arrest occasioned during a sporting activity was defined as one that occurred either in the course of the activity or within an hour of ceasing it.

I was surprised by how many out-of-hospital cardiac arrests there had been: 3,825, or more than one per 1,000. Of these, 2,144 occurred in a public space, and 2,070 were unrelated to sport. This left 74 cardiac arrests that occurred either during or within an hour of participation in sport. Of these, 16 occurred during competitive sports, and 58 during noncompetitive sporting activity such as jogging. Of the 74 cardiac arrests, 41 were fatal.

The proportion of the young population that indulged in competitive sports arranged or supervised by some kind of official organization was 11.4 percent. Of 352,499 persons, a third (116,390) played ice hockey. Only two of the cardiac arrests occurred among them by comparison with four among the 11,265 who played soccer. I leave it to statisticians to work out whether this means anything, or indeed could mean anything in the absence of control for factors such as age, social class, etc.

That cardiac arrests occur during or just after sporting activities does not mean that they were caused by those activities, of course: they might have occurred anyway. Oddly enough, this is a point the authors fail to make. In other studies, the rate of cardiac arrest in the general population of people between ages 12 and 45 has been estimated to be 4.84 per 100,000 per year, which means that even if sporting activity were the cause of cardiac arrests, they would cause only between a sixth and a seventh of them in this age group. On the other hand, sport is not the only form of vigorous physical exercise known to man, and the paper does not tell us what proportion of the 4.84 cardiac arrests per 100,000 per year occur in the midst of or just after vigorous exercise. Thus, we cannot exonerate physical exertion as a cause of cardiac arrest.

The authors naturally wanted to estimate what proportion of the deaths might have been prevented if medical examinations had been carried out on the athletes before they practiced their sport. (Not every athlete is athletic, of course.) In a sense, this inquiry was inherently unlikely to yield any practical results, for even if all 16 cardiac arrests (9 of them fatal) among the 352,499 sports participants were caused by detectable cardiac anomalies, screening procedures on nearly 40,000 people would, on average, prevent only a single death. In fact, the odds of doing good by screening are lower still, since most of the cardiac arrests occurred in people who had no identifiable illness or lesion beforehand. The authors estimate that screening 146,000 or more athletes would prevent only one cardiac arrest during sporting activity, and that screening 260,000 would prevent only one death.[1]

If sport were a pill, would doctors recommend it? I think not. We know that it causes many injuries, and cardiac arrest is not the only mode of death in sport. Chronic conditions such as osteoarthritis and dementia are also caused by sport. Any health benefits that sport might confer could be obtained by less vigorous exercise. That sport gives pleasure to millions cuts no ice with doctors of epidemiological bent (as we are all forced to be these days); smoking gives pleasure too, and I have never seen any reference to that pleasure in any medical literature about smoking, which refers only to tangible and measurable harms.

No, in a world ruled by doctors, there would be no sport.

One of the possible causes of cardiac arrest in sport is cardiomyopathy,

---

1 This assumes that sporting activity and cardiac arrests are causally related, which seems likely.

a progressive and inexorable deterioration of heart muscle, which, in the absence of a heart transplant, leads to death. Some types of cardiomyopathy are genetic in origin, and progress has recently been made in so-called gene editing, in which the replacement of the faulty causative gene with a healthier gene will be possible. Given the pace of technological development, this raises the specter of designer babies, of parents choosing the positive characteristics of their offspring and not just eliminating genetic defects.

Another article this week, however, calls attention to ethical difficulties of a more mundane but closely approaching nature. When genes in sperm or oocytes are edited it is not the parents who will be affected, but their offspring, and their offspring's offspring; and it cannot just be assumed that gene editing will produce only the desired effects and no others. The long-term effects of gene editing cannot be known in advance, and therefore there will have to be long-term follow-up studies on those who have been born gene-edited, as it were. But for these studies to be conducted, the consent of the subjects will have to be obtained, and it might not be forthcoming.

As the authors point out, the potential adverse effects of gene editing are disastrous, "even with small numbers of off-target edits." The subjects of the experiment were not party to the initial decision to participate, and they had no choice in the matter. I think I can hear in my mind's ear the rejoinder of a certain kind of bioethicist to this concern: After all, he would say, none of us asked to be born, and yet we were. Our parents involved us in a kind of natural experiment when they conceived us. Where, then, is the ethical difference or problem? True, the results of gene editing cannot be known in advance; but has this not been the case for natural conception for thousands of years?

What answer do we return? ◼

November 23, 2017

A re smartphones a blessing or a curse? When you are in a restaurant and observe four people around a table not speaking to one another, their eyes glued to the little screens, you think the phones are a curse, destructive of true social life and real human contact. Indeed, schools around the world are trying to reduce their distracting effects by prohibiting their use during the school day.

But that is not the whole story, of course, and in this week's *Journal* one can read of an ingenious, unexpected and unequivocally beneficial use of smartphones. Specifically, they are proving to be a highly useful and efficient tool in the campaign to eradicate river blindness in Africa. First, a little background is needed.

Onchocerciasis, or river blindness, is caused by a parasitic worm that goes by the charming name of *Onchocerca volvulus*. It is spread by the bite of little black flies, one of which goes by the equally grandiloquent name of *Simulium damnosum*. The flies breed in fast-flowing water.

A fertilized adult female *Onchocerca* worm, which lives up to fifteen years in its human host, produces tiny offspring, a thousand a day, called microfilariae. These pass into the *Simulium* fly when it—or rather she (the male of the species being vegetarian)—bites a person infected with the parasite. The microfilariae undergo development in the fly and eventually find their way into its saliva, by which they are transmitted back to a human host, where they migrate from the bloodstream to the skin tissue, where they mature into adult worms, and the whole process starts again. In a way, it is an admirable contrivance, though one wishes it could all have been to a better purpose.

Most of the microfilariae are not involved in reinfection (nature being wasteful of her progeny) and die in the human host, setting up an inflammatory reaction in the skin. If it occurs in the eye, it causes blindness. Onchocerciasis does not kill, but it blinds; it is the second commonest infective blindness in the world, now almost entirely confined to Africa.

There have been ongoing efforts to eradicate river blindness for more than forty years, and not even the most mystical of modern nature-worshipping pagans object to the attempted elimination of *Onchocerca volvulus* as a species.[1] Eradicating the disease can be done in two ways: via the fly or via the worm. Flies are more irrepressible than worms, however, and while initial efforts directed at *Simulium damnosum* appeared to be successful, the fly soon made a comeback. Fortunately, a drug was discovered that kills the microfilariae for about a year after ingestion; it is called ivermectin, and the discoverers were awarded a Nobel Prize in 2015. Ivermectin does not, alas, kill the adult worm that produces the microfilariae, but if everybody in an endemic area were to be treated once a year with ivermectin for fifteen years—the maximum life span of the worm—transmission of *Onchocerca* would be interrupted once and for all, and the disease eliminated.

Attempts at mass treatment with ivermectin were started, but unfortunately there was…I nearly said a fly in the ointment. In some areas, people were infected not only with *Onchocerca* but with another kind of filarial worm called *Loa loa*, which in adult form can live even longer in the human host, seventeen years. *Loa loa* is spread by another genus of flies, including *Chrysops silacea*. The worm causes an inflammatory reaction in the skin and can lead to very gross swellings; the adult worms move about and have a predilection for the eye. Infected people sometimes see a worm moving across their field of vision, and if it gets stuck there it has to be removed surgically. Incidentally, *Loa loa* does

---

1   There is a highly amusing webpage satirizing modern nature-worship or mysticism, http://www.deadlysins.com/guinea-worm, run by the shadowy Save the Guinea Worm Foundation, which is dedicated to opposing the eradication of another repellent parasite of humans that will soon be driven to extinction. The existence of such parasites is another example of the natural evil that theodicy is meant to explain, or (depending on your outlook) explain away.

not seem to have any host other than humans, so the worm and its life cycle must have evolved with man. If anyone ever tells you that man is no different from the other animals, you can reply, "Oh yes he is, he is susceptible to parasitization by *Loa loa*."

When ivermectin is given to people infected with *Loa loa*, a proportion of them suffer severe reactions and even die. *Loa loa* produces vastly greater numbers of microfilariae than does *Onchocerca*, and ivermectin duly kills them; but where they are extremely numerous, more than 30,000 per cubic millimeter of blood, their death may set up a severe and sometimes fatal inflammatory reaction around the brain. In a mass campaign of treatment with ivermectin in 1999 in an area of Cameroon, 500 people suffered from encephalitis, from which 60 died. Understandably, ivermectin was not used there again—until 2015, but with a new strategy.

The article in this week's *Journal* relates how doctors and researchers returned to the same area of Cameroon to perform a new mass campaign with ivermectin. This time, before giving it to anyone, they checked the *Loa loa* filarial count in his blood, and they refrained from giving the drug to anyone with a count higher than 26,000 per cubic millimeter.

Participation in the campaign was impressive, given the persisting memory of the earlier one: 16,259 of 22,842 persons living in the area (71.2 percent) agreed to take part. Everyone who participated was treated except those who had too high a filarial count, or were in poor general health, or were pregnant or inebriated (what a humanizing picture that single word in the middle of a scientific paper conjures up!). All together, 737 people (4.4 percent of the population surveyed) were excluded, and of the remaining 15,552 people, 22 percent had onchocerciasis. No person treated had a serious reaction to the drug as in the previous campaign, and none died.

What really astonished me, however, was the manner in which the counts of *Loa loa* microfilaria in the blood were established. This is where smartphones enter the story:

> The LoaScope, a mobile-telephone-based videomicrosope…was developed. With the use of a smartphone coupled to a simple optical device, the LoaScope automatically counts *L. loa* microfilariae in peripheral blood collected in disposable rectangular capillary tubes without the need for sample processing.

How admirable—more than admirable—the ingenuity, and this time to what a worthy end! The people who used the LoaScope were trained in its use in an hour. This means it should be possible, in theory, to reduce the prevalence of onchocerciasis to very low levels and perhaps, with the addition of *Simulium* control, to eliminate it entirely. Of course, the price of onchocerciasis elimination is, if not eternal vigilance exactly, vigilance for fifteen years.

Even rural Africa now has telephone networks. (When I was in Africa, phoning anyone more than a few hundred yards away was a labor of Hercules, and often not possible at all, especially in the rainy season.) And notwithstanding the supposed legacy of colonialism so fondly emphasized in a thousand academic publications, the people of the area must have placed a considerable degree of trust in the interlopers who came to help them.

〜

As we have just seen, not all the works of nature are benign from the human point of view. Not many of us are fond of slugs—least of all, gardeners; and while for some of us a rose may be a rose may be a rose, for most of us quite definitely a slug is a slug is a slug. Recently, however, I bought a book by a slug enthusiast in the hope of repairing my lamentable ignorance of these creatures. While most books about slugs teach you how to kill them, this one tells you how to preserve them. I have not yet gone this far.

Are slugs of medical interest? This week's article in the *NEJM* series "Clinical Implications of Medical Research" discusses the mucus-based multicomponent glue that the dusky arion slug (*Arion subfuscus*) secretes when under threat. The secretion makes it difficult for predators to dislodge the slug.

Looking into the composition of this glue, researchers have developed a similar glue which they hope might serve as an adhesive in surgical operations, where sutures and metal clips have many disadvantages. This all strikes me again as admirably clever: first the observation of the secretion, then the leap of the imagination to think that it might have some useful application, then the elucidation of its structure, and finally the development of a synthetic analogue. What a piece of work is a man—and a slug, come to that. ▪

November 30, 2017

The current epidemic of opioid overdose in the United States does not reflect well on at least a portion of the medical profession, whose sloppy, thoughtless and in some cases corrupt prescription habits contributed considerably to its development. Even now, if my acquaintances are anything to go by, doctors are willing to prescribe opioids to postoperative patients who do not need them, and in quantities that would addict or even kill a village. Since my acquaintances are sensible and decent, they flush the pills down the lavatory rather than ingest them or sell them, but it is as if the doctors prescribing them had not heard the news for the last year or two.[1]

It is likely that the role of doctors in causing the epidemic has declined, and the torch, so to speak, has been taken up by private enterprise in the form of drug smugglers and dealers, who have seized the opportunity to grow their business (to use the inelegant language of the management books sold at airport bookstands).

A case report in the *NEJM* series called "Case Records of the Massachusetts General Hospital" recounts the story of a 36-year-old man who was found deeply unconscious in a park on a winter's afternoon. The signs and symptoms were suggestive of an opioid overdose. He was found by a friend, who administered naloxone, the antidote to opioid overdose, and called the emergency services, who brought him to

---

1 Both the American news media and the medical profession were lamentably slow to react to a situation that had obviously been developing over nearly two decades.

hospital. There he was administered more naloxone and, being found to have pulmonary edema, was also give diuretics and oxygen. He made an uneventful recovery, and denied having had any intention to overdose. In other words, he supposed that he was taking only a "normal" (that is to say, *his* normal) dose of opioids. Certainly, his friend must have been *au fait* with the complications of drug abuse.

Chemical examination of his urine revealed no opioids, but it was conducted rather late, by which time the metabolites tested for would have disappeared, and the tests would not in any case have detected the presence of fentanyl, the synthetic opioid, much stronger than morphine or heroin, that is increasingly used to "cut" those drugs. The degree to which this is done with illicit supplies varies, so that the addict does not know what he is taking. Severe overdose may result from taking what he mistakenly supposes to be his "normal" dose, which is what appears to have happened in this case.

The article is less detailed in its account than one would hope. According to the medical history provided here, the patient had been taking opioids for four years before this episode:

> Approximately 4 years before this evaluation the patient had under-gone an unspecified hand surgery. Immediately after the procedure hydromorphone was administered. After the patient was discharged home he initially sought out more prescription opioids and then switched to intravenous heroin because he found it to be less expensive and more readily obtained. During the next 3 years he injected 1 to 2 g. [grams] of heroin each day.

This account is somewhat schematic, to say the least. First, we are not informed of its source. However, the fact that the hand surgery which supposedly started his slide into addiction was "unspecified" suggests that the account is taken from the patient, and not from any contemporaneous record, for no such record would just say "hand surgery—unspecified." Nor are we told how long he was hospitalized, or for how long the hydromorphone "was administered." It is unlikely that he spent more than a day or two in hospital, given the (sometimes unseemly) eagerness with which patients are discharged these days. He could not possibly have developed hydromorphone addiction while he was there. He "sought out more prescription opioids" after his discharge, which suggests that his surgeons did not suppose that his postoperative pain would be very severe. It also suggests that his addiction was the result of what he did rather than what others did to him or something that just crept up on him like a thief in the night. As to his "switch to intravenous heroin," it too was active rather than passive. As all such addicts do, he had quite a lot to learn, if he didn't know it already: where to get heroin, how to prepare it, where to get his needles and syringes, how to inject the drug, how to overcome the normal inhibition against sticking a needle into himself. Contrary to popular belief, addiction to opioids is not instantaneous, nor does it imply an inexorable fate when it happens, or is achieved.

The discussion of this case is naive, or perhaps gives the impression of naivety because of its attachment to *bien pensant* notions. The man is said to have suffered from *opioid-use disorder*; it cannot be called *abuse* any longer. (But if it is only use and not abuse, why should it be called a disorder?) The implied evidence tells us that this man brought the addiction upon himself, but such a view of addiction is nowadays castigated as stigmatizing. There is an underlying assumption that if he brought the problem upon himself, he would deserve no help. Since we want to help him, however, he could not have brought it upon himself. But if we were to deny assistance to all those who brought problems upon themselves, we should help only a very restricted portion of mankind.

The writers of this case lament the absence of facilities to help such men as this, though they provide evidence that he had several times refused assistance. When finally he accepted it, he reported that he had managed not to take heroin for six months.[2] This, incidentally, illustrates how difficult it is to establish whether any "treatment" for such an addiction really works. By the time an addict is ready to cooperate with it, he has already changed his mind. The fact that addicts quite often give up drugs following a religious conversion suggests that "treatment" is not straightforwardly pharmacological or physiological—except, perhaps, for strict mind-brain identity theorists.

---

2 The authors credited his report, which might or might not have been true.

Advance end-of-life directives are often assumed to be a good thing, and doctors are fond of quoting the lines from Arthur Hugh Clough's "The Latest Decalogue" in precisely the opposite sense from that which he intended:

> Thou must not kill, but needst not strive
> Officiously to keep alive.

That doctors get it precisely wrong is obvious from all the other couplets, such as:

> Thou shalt not steal; an empty feat
> When 'tis so lucrative to cheat.

A letter in this week's *Journal* describes a case in which a 70-year-old patient with diabetes, chronic bronchitis or emphysema and atrial fibrillation arrived unconscious in hospital. Across his chest were tattooed the words *DO NOT RESUSCITATE*. Should the doctors try to save his life or not? His condition suggested a life that had not been lived healthily. He had a high alcohol level in his blood, and his lung condition half-implied a lifetime of heavy smoking in bars.[3]

The doctors called for an urgent consultation from ethicists. (The very existence of such "ethics consultants" seems to me an attempt to divide responsibility for making hard decisions so that *no one* is ultimately responsible for them, just as firing squads have at least one among them who is given a blank.) The ethicists, as I would have predicted, thought the tattoo ought to be taken *au sérieux* rather than as something done in a drunken state.

The doctors made no attempt to save the man, and he duly died. Rather chillingly, the authors say:

> Subsequently, the social work department obtained a copy of his Florida Department of Health "out-of-hospital" DNR [Do Not Resuscitate] order, which was consistent with the tattoo.

---

3 Most people who turn up drunk in hospitals are heavy drinkers, if not alcoholics.

The authors, I suspect, suffered from a certain degree of unease, for on a first reading of their letter it is not entirely clear whether *subsequently* means subsequent to the ethicists' advice but before the patient was allowed to die, or subsequent to his death. Almost certainly, the latter is meant.

For myself, I can only hope that just before my death I fall into the hands of humane doctors of sound judgment—their own judgment, that is. ◾

December 7, 2017

However many times we are warned that correlation is not causation, there is something in the human mind that resists the warning. No sooner is a statistical correlation established, or at least asserted, than we think we know a cause. When, some years ago, publicity was given to a study that showed a correlation between low selenium levels and heart attacks, there was a run on brazil nuts in supermarkets such that they were soon nowhere to be found, because brazil nuts are of high selenium content. The increasing prevalence of epidemiological studies encourages us to go from correlation to correlation, as bees go from flower to flower, in our efforts to distill from them the honey of a healthy life and therefore of longevity, if not immortality.

The founding father of epidemiological studies, Austin Bradford Hill, in 1965 laid down some principles—now often ignored in practice—to estimate whether or not a correlation implied causation. These principles are rules of thumb rather than binding laws, and their precise epistemological status is ambiguous. They are as follows:

1. The higher the correlation, the more likely it indicates causation, though a weak correlation does not automatically mean that the relationship is not causative.
2. The correlation should be reproducible.
3. The more specific the population and its circumstances, the more likely is any correlation within it to be causative.

4. The effect must occur after the cause, though delay does not preclude causation.

5. There should be a dose-response relationship between the supposed cause and the effect, such that a lower exposure to the cause should result in a lower incidence.

6. The relationship between proposed cause and effect should be biologically plausible, though of course the current state of ignorance may make a causative relationship seem implausible.

7. There should be agreement between epidemiological and other forms of evidence.

8. Ideally, experimental evidence should support a causative relationship.

9. Analogy with other similar instances is suggestive though not probative.

With these principles in mind, I read an epidemiological paper in this week's *Journal* titled "Contemporary Hormonal Contraception and the Risk of Breast Cancer." The authors address the thorny question whether those women who use, or have ever used, hormonal contraception are more at risk of breast cancer than those who have not. Some studies have shown that there is no increased risk, but others have shown the opposite. I suppose every investigator wants the last word on a matter of controversy, to settle it once and for all.

The paper comes from Denmark, and once again one is torn between admiration of a system that enables access to every person's health record in the country, and a slight feeling of unease that there is no escape from the state's benevolence—or malevolence, if things should turn that way. Be that all as it may, it is a matter of astonishment that a country with so small a population relative to others is nevertheless able to conduct epidemiological studies on a scale difficult or impossible in other, much larger countries. The National Register of Medicinal Product Statistics had complete data on all prescriptions in Denmark as of January 1, 1995, so that was used as the starting date of the study period.

The authors examined—electronically, of course—the medical records of every single woman in Denmark who was between the ages of 15 and 49 on that date, and additionally those who reached the age of 15 by December 31, 2012: a total of 1,837,297 women. After a relatively few exclusions for intercurrent illnesses that would have interfered with the results, the records of 1,797,932 women (over a period of nearly 11 years on average) were examined for their use of hormonal contraceptives and their development of cancer. Again, it is a matter of astonishment that the authors, thanks to the Danish system, were able to trace every prescription for hormonal contraceptives that had been filled in the country between 1995 and 2012.

In essence, what they found was that women who had used hormonal contraceptives had a 20 percent higher rate of breast cancer than those who had never used one. This means that there is one extra case of breast cancer for every 9,690 women who use such a contraceptive for a year.[1]

This is surely unfortunate for the one woman in 9,690, but is the overall risk anything worth worrying about? A friend of mine, a distinguished professor, says that he takes no notice of a risk so small; that until the odds ratio reaches 2—when the risk in the experimental group is twice that of the control—it is essentially a form of epidemiological white noise. I think this is a little brusque or too summary; but let us set aside the question for a moment and look at another one: is the observed relationship a causative one?

The authors found a clear gradient between the length of exposure to hormonal contraceptives and the additional risk. This in itself does not prove causation, since some other factor, acting simultaneously, could also have caused the increasing risk. But it does nevertheless fulfill one of the Austin Bradford Hill criteria.

Women in the study used hormonal contraceptives not only for differing lengths of time, but also in different preparations, containing different hormones. The authors were able to find no differences according to the preparations used, which I find slightly disconcerting, at least on the hypothesis of a causative relationship. Is it likely that *all* preparations were equally carcinogenic? On the other hand, large though the sample was, perhaps it was not large enough to pick up statistically significant differences between the risks associated with using different preparations.

---

1 Or, on the assumption that the relationship between the length of exposure and risk is linear (which it isn't), one in 969 for those who use hormonal contraception for ten years.

Another finding that is possibly in keeping with a causative relationship is that, though an increased risk persists for five years after stopping the treatment, it declines thereafter (as the risks associated with smoking decline though do not disappear after cessation). On the other hand, the authors did not—could not—control for other important possible factors, such as the number of children the women had borne, or obesity. They rather airily dismiss such factors, claiming that they would have to be very strong to make the correlation between hormonal contraception and cancer disappear; but of course there might be several of them, bringing their seasoning to the cauldron of causation.

Is the study reproducible? In its exact form, probably not; and one of the problems with this kind of work is that it frequently produces different results. As the authors say, "Studies of breast-cancer risk among women who receive hormonal contraceptives show inconsistent findings—from no elevation in risk to a 20 to 30% increase in risk."

Altogether, though I am no expert, the paper seems to me less than overwhelmingly convincing, but an accompanying editorial commenting on it says, "these data suggest that the search for an oral contraceptive that does not elevate the risk of breast cancer needs to continue." The author of the editorial thus accepts that the relationship is a causative one; that correlation in this case *is* cause.

One of the striking omissions in this paper is the exclusion of death rates, both from cancer and all causes, from its analysis. This would be useful information, since false positive diagnoses of breast cancer are common. Because hormonal contraception has often been suspected of being a cause of breast cancer, people on such contraception might be examined more frequently for breast cancer: seek and ye shall find, though it is known that some of what is found is spurious.

How complicated the world is!

꧁

Austin Bradford Hill was also one of the founding fathers of the controlled trial as a means of obtaining true medical knowledge. But controlled trials are not everything, and it is possible to achieve advances without them. In a startling and inspiring paper on hemophilia B, we learn that ten patients were given one-time therapy with a gene for producing an effective form of the clotting factor that they lacked, a lack that resulted in dangerous and painful bleeding episodes. Over a follow-up period of a year, it was found that the infusion of this gene reduced their bleeding episodes and in most cases eliminated them altogether. They no longer needed infusions of the clotting factor every few days or when they started bleeding.

This is a remarkable triumph of scientific medicine. The point I wish to make here, however, is that the results of this trial were impressive even though the trial did not meet the modern canons of controlled experiment. There were no controls, except as far as the patients were their own controls. Before treatment, horrible symptoms; after treatment, no horrible symptoms. It is almost inconceivable that anything other than the treatment could have produced this result.

Evidence should be of a type appropriate to the matter under investigation. This is obvious but is sometimes forgotten. ▣

December 14, 2017

We have already seen that repeated admonitions that correlation is not to be confused with causation do not seem to have much effect, and in like fashion warnings against our natural propensity to seek blame when things go wrong fall on deaf ears. The fact is that affixing blame is enjoyable in a way that merely finding causes is not. It reassures us that whatever happens is under human control. Moreover, just as correlation sometimes *is* an indication of cause, so in some cases blame is justified. We do not have to go quite as far as the Azande of the Sudan, who—as described by the social anthropologist E. E. Evans-Pritchard—believed that every death was caused by the malign magic of the enemies of the deceased, but we *can* acknowledge that some deaths are blameworthy (which is why medical malpractice takes the place of malign magic in some people's minds).

The problem is that culpability is often diffuse, rather than attachable to one easily identified scapegoat. In such circumstances, however, a general principle may be discerned: sue the culprit with the most money. There is no point in suing a pauper, however much to blame he might be.

One of the two articles in this week's *Journal* dealing with the epidemic of death by overdose of opioids in the United States looks rather like an instance of fixing blame where the money is. (The *NEJM* was not very quick off the mark to recognize the scale of the problem— now some 300,000 deaths since the turn of the millennium—but it can no longer be accused of neglecting the issue.) In "Drug Companies' Liability for the Opioid Epidemic," the two authors, both of them lawyers by training,[1] more or less start from the premise that the drug companies who manufactured the newer semisynthetic opioids such as hydromorphone and oxycontin are legally and morally liable, and ought to be sued as much and as often as possible.

I have no particular sympathy for the drug companies: it is beyond reasonable doubt that they used high-pressure tactics and dishonest salesmanship to induce doctors to prescribe their products inappropriately. But twenty years into the epidemic, it is surely rather feeble to blame them, except in the sense that Eve was responsible for all of mankind's subsequent woes.

The article points out that early attempts to sue the companies for personal injury faced considerable obstacles. If, for example, the companies failed to provide proper warnings in their product information, what are we to say of the licensing agency, the FDA, which licensed the products *as they were in fact marketed*? Furthermore, as the authors point out, "juries may resist laying legal responsibility at the manufacturer's feet when the prescriber's decisions and the patient's behavior contributed to the harm."

In order to "overcome" any inclination of jurors to think that individuals might have some responsibility for their behavior, the authors recommend the "procedural strategy" of filing a class action suit:

> In such suits, the causal relationship between the companies' business model and the harm is assessed at the group level, with the focus on statistical associations between product use and injury. The use of class actions was instrumental in overcoming tobacco companies' defenses based on smokers' conduct.

How delightful for lawyers, but how sinister from the point of view of natural justice! It would mean that an individual's culpability for a misdeed shrinks as the number of people committing the same misdeed grows. The larger the mob, the smaller the sin.

This is not the place to criticize in any detail this kind of morally, intellectually and financially corrupt litigation. Suffice it to say that the principal beneficiaries of the tobacco litigation were the lawyers who

---

1 Everyone's vested interests are easy to discern but one's own.

brought it (who, of course, did not wish to drive the companies into bankruptcy, for they wanted to sue those companies again and again); and that the principal beneficiaries, by far, of tobacco sales have long been governments, which have the power to restrict or even forbid sales but have not used it.

What if governments were to stand as injured parties and bring lawsuits themselves? The authors propose this strategy with respect to opioids:

> Perhaps the most promising development in opioid litigation has been the advent of suits brought against drug makers and distributors by the federal government and dozens of states. . . . Because the government itself is claiming injury and seeking restitution so that it can repair social systems debilitated by opioid addiction, these suits avoid defenses that blame opioid consumers or prescribers. They also garner substantial publicity.

Again, there is not space enough to comment on this in anything like the detail it deserves. Let us just consider some of the unexamined premises: a) that the money obtained by the government will be used to "repair social systems debilitated by opioid addiction"; b) that the government can identify and isolate "social systems" and then "repair" them; and c) that the opioid addiction was a cause of the debilitation of social systems rather than a manifestation of it.[2] But most important, this litigation makes a distant cause, or alleged cause, more liable than a proximate one, purely (I surmise) for the reason that the distant cause can be litigated more profitably than the proximate one.

Moreover, this article is reminiscent of the Red Queen's kind of justice: sentence first, verdict afterward. Running through the article is the supposition that the drug companies' defenses are not really defenses at all, but merely sophistical obstacles to be overcome. The end (the "repair of social systems") justifies the means. The authors, be it noted, teach at prestigious institutions. Though I despise what the principal company involved actually did, I find this unsettling.

---

2 In fact, the relationship is likely to have been *dialectical*, to employ a frequently abused word.

∽

A second article on the opioid crisis deals with attempts to change doctors' prescribing habits (a tacit admission that they have something important to do with the causation of the epidemic). In Massachusetts, one of the states worst affected by the epidemic, the state government sent notices to doctors informing them whether they prescribed more or less opioid medication than their peers. Once they were armed with this information, their prescribing habits (in aggregate) changed hardly at all.

There was more than one possible reason for this, which the authors of the article do not mention. The first is that the doctors did not actually read the information provided to them. There must surely be some law of declining marginal effect of circulated information to doctors (and others, of course). Certainly, when I was in practice my eyes tended to glaze over very quickly when I received circulars, usually written in a style that was to prose what wet chewing gum is to the soles of shoes. Circulars were seldom a pleasure to read.

The second possible (unmentioned) reason is that doctors like to imagine that their practice is impeccable, that what they do is the acme of good sense, prudence and benevolence. In theory, and occasionally if reluctantly in practice, we are open to correction. But the notion that others do things in a better way than we do meets with resistance and provokes an *I'll show 'em* reaction in us. If we change our practice, it is a virtual admission that we have been doing things wrong, which is not an easy admission to make, especially if our actions may have resulted in death.

The authors do suggest that the information provided may have acted as a stimulus for low prescribers to prescribe more, as much as for high prescribers to prescribe less. If it had both effects, they would cancel each other out, and the aggregate would remain the same (as it did). I was reminded of a reeducation course that I was encouraged to take—by the abrogation of punishment—after I was caught speeding. The policeman who ran the course pointed out that speed limits were *limits*, not targets. Oddly enough, I had never thought of this before: I had always thought of them as targets, to be exceeded if possible.

The authors, who seem to have made health-care policy and management rather than clinical care the focus of their careers, claim that "there is a real danger that aggressive opioid-prescribing policies could…force patients to live with inadequately treated pain." I think this demonstrates that the authors have not grasped the true dimension or nature of the scandal, namely, that the opioid medications from which so many people have died were always ineffective in the relief of the pain for which they were prescribed, and should never have been prescribed in the first place. This is an inglorious episode in the history of medicine. ◪

December 21, 2017

One of the formative experiences of my intellectual development was hearing a lecture by Professor Thomas McKeown and subsequently reading a book of his, *The Role of Medicine: Dream, Mirage or Nemesis?* (1976). McKeown was a professor of social medicine who helped to puncture the medical profession's deep self-regard, and replace it by a more skeptical modesty.

At the time I heard McKeown speak, one of medicine's greatest historical achievements was the discovery of the cause of tuberculosis and subsequently of an effective treatment for it: streptomycin, which first went on the U.S. market in 1946 and became available in Britain soon afterward. (If George Orwell had not been untreatably allergic to streptomycin, he might well have lived into the 1980s or even beyond.)

Doctors easily and unquestioningly believed that the precipitous decline in the incidence of tuberculosis had been due to their efforts, a belief which was flattering to their self-esteem. But McKeown showed that the decline in the death rate from tuberculosis, from its peak in the middle of the nineteenth century, was precipitous even before the bacteriological cause or any genuine therapy had been found. The smooth gradient of the decline showed a line uninterrupted by any medical discovery at any point from 1850 to 1950, and therefore something other than medical progress had to explain it. The explanation that McKeown offered was that of improved social conditions, including nutrition and housing.

In fact, Rudolf Virchow (1821–1902), the founder of cellular pathology, had warned against the simplistic monocausal view of tuberculosis. At the height of tuberculosis's command as Captain of the Men of Death, practically every person was exposed to the germ that caused it; but even then, only a minority of persons went on to develop the disease. In other words, the tuberculous bacillus was a necessary but not a sufficient cause of the disease. Virchow, though principally a pathologist, was a strong campaigner for sanitary reform.

But the truth is yet more complex than the equation *Bad social conditions plus tuberculous bacillus equals tuberculosis.* There is still individual variation, and I discovered on some Pacific islands where I worked an exceptionally high rate of tuberculosis, not only of the lungs but of the spine, abdomen, cervical glands, pericardium and kidneys. It is true that the islands were poor in monetary income, but they offered a generous subsistence economy and, thanks to an even and almost unvarying climate, a healthy outdoor lifestyle of a kind one would not normally have thought of as propitious to tuberculosis. And yet tuberculosis was rampant there.

Why? The most obvious explanation was that the population had not yet been sifted by the harsh sorting methods of evolution. Tuberculosis was unknown in the islands before the arrival of the Europeans and therefore the population had not had generations to select the types most resistant to it. Insofar as there is a genetic susceptibility to the disease, the islanders were most susceptible.

Partly in response to overconfidence in the promise of genetic science to solve medical problems, a paper in this week's *Journal* takes up the hoary and contentious subject of whether medicine and doctors treat diseases or whole persons or societies. Under the title "Putting the Patient Back Together—Social Medicine, Network Medicine, and the Limits of Reductionism," the authors present a schematic history of modern medicine, according to which its first phase was the sorting of diseases into valid natural types as a prerequisite for building a rational basis for therapeutics. In the second phase, gross pathology (the study of pathology on a macroscopic scale) was developed. In the third, pathology went microscopic. Then came the germ theory of disease,[1] followed by the biochemical and genomic phases.

---

1 Such luminaries as George Bernard Shaw never accepted the germ theory, regarding it as a hoax or a fraud.

The authors say that the potential benefits of the Human Genome Project were grossly oversold, and perhaps this should have been known in advance. In a sense, the hyperbole represented a regression to pre-Virchowian thought, the idea that disease is a monocausal phenomenon—the single cause now being a faulty gene. In fact, however, even where diseases are caused by mutations in a single gene, their expression in clinical disease is variable, from unnoticeable to extremely severe and life-threatening. Even here, disease does not always have a single sufficient cause, and other contributory causes must be found.

Against this history, the article is yet another appeal for doctors to treat that evasive entity, the Whole Person. This is not an isolated creature, a particle in Brownian motion, but rather a social being whose environment, both physical and social, profoundly affects his health. It is known that lonely people, for example, are more susceptible to many kinds of disease. It has also been proposed that the current epidemic of obesity is caused by social emulation: people become fat by being around fat people.[2] The doctor, then must treat more than necessary causes of disease, but the Whole Person.

In a sense, this is another instance of the higher cliché. Every sensible and experienced doctor has always known that disease is often not simply a matter of a single exciting cause. And yet there is no doubt also that doctors placed extravagant and unrealistic hopes in the Human Genome Project. As the article puts it,

> The hyperbole surrounding the Human Genome Project encouraged the scientific community and the public to believe that simple knowledge of genomic variation would—in a linear, reductionist way—inform us about disease susceptibility and lead to individual treatments.[3] Both the media and leaders in genomics perpetuated this myth, the latter cataloguing genomic variants associated with complex disease phenotypes as if these lists formed a Rosetta Stone of disease causation.

---

2 Another possible interpretation of the social clustering of the fat is that birds of a feather flock together.

3 It has done so, but rarely, and certainly not to the extent of changing the conditions of human existence very much for most of us.

The very fact that calls for treating the Whole Person are frequently recurrent puts me in mind of what the Spanish colonial officials used to say on receiving royal instructions from the metropolis: *Obedezco pero no cumplo*, "I obey but do not fulfill." Such calls are often expressed in high-flown incantatory phraseology, for lack of any concrete proposal. The conclusion of this article is an example:

> The task of putting the patient back together again will be complex, arduous, and time consuming, but it promises a new articulation of the biologic and social sciences that are inextricably linked and essential to the advancement of medicine.

Let us now turn to the latest case record of the Massachusetts General Hospital published in the *Journal* to see how the pious wish expressed is complied with. The case is of a 41-year-old woman who had recurrent chest pain. Her social situation was assessed only insofar as it might reveal risk factors for certain diseases that may have caused her chest pain: did she smoke, for example, or take cocaine? But otherwise the assessment was purely biomechanical. She underwent a series of sophisticated tests mainly to assess the condition of her heart, especially concentrating on the coronary arteries. It was discovered eventually that she had had what is called dissection of the coronary artery: the inner and outer layer of the artery become separated after a tear of the inner layer allows blood to flow between them.

In this case, the woman had relatives with Ehlers-Danlos syndrome, a disorder of connective tissue that predisposes to dissections of arteries. She therefore underwent genetic testing to discern whether she had that condition, or one like it. If she did, any further child she might bear would have a 50 percent chance of inheriting the disease. (She already had an 11-year-old daughter, who was healthy.) Testing showed that the woman did not have the syndrome.

She did not require much in the way of treatment. Apart from a few initial questions about her habits and way of life, her case was treated as a purely biomechanical problem. There was no need for a Whole Person approach, and in this respect the case was a perfectly straightforward one. It would have been very different if, for instance, the patient had suffered from spasm of the coronary artery brought about by abuse of cocaine. A more holistic treatment might then have been appropriate, though whether it would have been crowned with success is another matter. ◾

December 28, 2017

We take the safety of our medicines for granted, at least in the sense that they will not contain gross impurities; side effects are another thing entirely. We assume that medicines are what they say on the packet that they are. We forget that this has not always been the case, nor is it the case in many places in the world today. In Nigeria, for example, up to 50 percent of medicines sold are counterfeit, and some of the forgeries show considerable sophistication, worthy of a better object. In the hospital in which I worked, patients were sometimes treated for lead or arsenic poisoning that contaminated ayurvedic medicines. No doubt accidents sometimes happen in the manufacturing process, and it has even been known for psychopaths to contaminate production lines of drugs with the intention of poisoning as many people as possible; but the purity of our medicine supply is surely an unsung achievement. Progress is taken for granted the moment it is made, and people forget that things were ever otherwise.

There have been some exceptions to this achievement in recent years, however, and the problem arises primarily when drugs need extra compounding (preparation) for people to be able to take them. It may be that the numbers of people who require a special preparation of a drug, such as a liquid formulation because of difficulties with swallowing, are not large enough for it to be worthwhile for pharmaceutical companies to make it in that form. The drug then has to be sent to a compounding center to be liquefied.

In 2012, as an article in this week's *Journal* recounts, the New

England Compounding Center (a private facility) sent a batch of con-taminated methylprednisolone injections all over the country. As a result, 750 people suffered fungal meningitis, and 64 of them died. The article does not mention that both the owner and the chief pharmacist of the offending company were sentenced to nine years' imprisonment. Nor does it mention one of the most tragic aspects of the episode: that there is little evidence of the drug's efficacy as an injection to treat low back pain, which is how it was being used.

The article is written by employees of the Food and Drug Administration, and perhaps not surprisingly it omits to mention that, at the time, the FDA was blamed for (which is not quite the same as saying it was guilty of) not having prevented the outbreak, since the violations of safety procedures by the company had been repeated and longstanding. The FDA argued in its defense that its jurisdiction in the case was unclear at the time and therefore it was inhibited in its actions.

The FDA's powers were then clarified and strengthened—a case of shutting the stable door after the horse has bolted, which is an inevitable process in human affairs, for we often learn by disaster. Subsequently there have been other cases of mal-compounding of medications, none with quite such catastrophic consequences, though some bad enough. Of 425 inspections of compounding facilities since 2012, the FDA inspectors found "problematic conditions" in the great majority:

> Examples of observations include dead insects in compounding areas designated for sterile compounding, visible mold on ceiling tiles in compounding rooms, and dog beds and dog hairs in close proximity to compounding areas.

The price of purity is eternal vigilance, but vigilance drives up prices.

The effect of competition on the price of generic prescription drugs is examined in a letter to the *Journal*. The authors compared the prices of such drugs with the prices of brand-name drugs, and then plotted the relative generic-to-brand prices, in percentages, against the number of manufacturers that produced generic versions of the drug. The results were clear, at least graphically (though their meaning is another thing).

When there was only one company that made a generic version of a drug, the price was similar to the brand-name version, though of course somewhat lower (87 percent) in order to provide sufficient incentive to buyers. The more manufacturers in the field, the lower the price: if there were two manufacturers, the price dropped to 77 percent of the brand-name price; if there were five manufacturers, the price went down to 46 percent; and with ten or more manufacturers, the price was 21 percent. The effect of competition seems plain enough.

But is it really quite so straightforward? What determines the number of manufacturers in the field in the first place? It must surely depend to a considerable extent on the size of the market for the drug, the costs and difficulty of manufacture, and so forth; and these factors would complicate the relationship between number of manufacturers and price. (The authors of the letter cautiously, and wisely, titled it "Prices of Generic Drugs Associated with Numbers of Manufacturers," rather than asserting a cause-and-effect relationship between those variables.)

When it comes to pharmaceutical policy, if I may so call it, we have at least two desiderata that are incompatible. The first is that there should be as much innovation as possible; the second is that whatever is produced should be perfectly safe. But safety considerations raise the costs of innovation and entry into the market. In practice, we choose security rather than innovation—or rather "we" as a society so choose, since we have little individually to do with the choice. This suits regulators, of course, for it not only provides them with employment but also simplifies their work. As for the giant pharmaceutical companies, it suits them very well too, for it is more comfortable to work in a cartelized environment than in a truly competitive one.

This issue of the *Journal* contains a paper on the treatment of patients with hemophilia A by gene transfer, and it might be regarded as more important than the one published three issues ago on gene therapy for hemophilia B. This is because hemophilia A is five or six times more common than hemophilia B, and because hemophilia A was hitherto believed to be inherently the more difficult to treat by gene therapy (for reasons that I do not fully understand, but which relate to the size of the gene that has to be replaced).

Seven people were treated, and the results were similar to those published for hemophilia B. One year after a single infusion of the replacement gene, episodes of bleeding and the need for infusion of the blood factor that is missing in hemophilia A were enormously reduced in all patients. These results hold out the hope of a normal existence for those who suffer from this disease. It is hard not to be profoundly impressed by this work.

But then a horrible thought entered my mind, like a worm in the bud. This work is grossly unjust. The expense of the experiment (conducted in London) was almost certainly enormous. Such expense probably precludes the work from being applied to large numbers of people very rapidly. It is true, of course, that there is a tendency for the cost of any treatment to come down as it becomes routine, but this inevitably takes some time. For the foreseeable future, the gene therapy that has had so dramatic a beneficial effect on the lives of the seven people so far treated will not be available to the vast majority of sufferers from hemophilia A. Where is the justice in that? By what criteria could a small elite of patients be chosen? In a commercial system it would be by ability to pay; in any other system it would be arbitrary, by place of residence, on a first come first served basis, or perhaps by an estimate of the increase in the number of "quality-adjusted life-years" that any suffering individuals might expect as a result of the treatment. What is certain, however, is that the treatment for now can only increase inequalities in the life experience of hemophiliacs, inequalities that are arbitrarily distributed and therefore unjust. Indeed, even if all the hemophiliacs in any country could be treated equally, this would still not reduce the injustice associated with the treatment, at least until all hemophiliacs in the world had equal access to the treatment.

In the name of justice, therefore, it is imperative that all research that could benefit patients differentially—which is to say, *all* research— should cease forthwith. ◼

January 4, 2018

The precautionary principle is what now rules the world, including that small corner of it that is the practice of medicine. Probably more prescriptions are issued worldwide on the basis of the precautionary principle than are issued to treat actual illnesses that are known to patients by the symptoms they currently experience. For example, many millions of people are prescribed medication for high blood pressure, a symptomless disease (except in its most malignant form, which is rare). Most people who take this medication are probably under the misapprehension that it will do them good, when in fact it is very unlikely to do them good, and more likely to do them harm. That harm will probably be slight, in side effects, while the good it might do them (with perhaps a one in a hundred chance over five years that it will) is considerable: preventing a heart attack or a stroke. A distinguished clinical pharmacologist friend of mine thinks that not one in a hundred people on such treatment understands the purpose for it; he thinks it might be one in two hundred who do.[1]

The precautionary principle is applicable—or is applied, at any rate—when the possibility of an adverse outcome is suspected but the precise degree of risk is unknown. The adverse outcome, while as yet purely imaginary, is often more present in people's minds than the actual harm done in the present to avoid it. In a way, this is opposed (though

---

1 This raises an important question about informed consent. Is what counts the information given by the doctor, or the information absorbed, understood and retained by the patient?

not diametrically) to the distinction, made famous by the nineteenth-century French liberal economist Frédéric Bastiat,[2] between what is seen and not seen, in which a policy to right an immediate problem causes unforeseen (but foreseeable) problems in the future.

A case could be made that it was Pythagoras who first applied the precautionary principle, when he enjoined his followers to abjure beans—broad beans of the *Vicia faba* plant—as if they were disgusting, and avoiding them a moral duty. Pythagoras makes an appearance in a review article about a condition known as *favism*, a form of hemolytic anemia caused in part by the consumption of beans.[3]

Favism occurs in people who have a genetic deficiency of an enzyme called glucose-6-phosphate dehydrogenase. This deficiency makes it impossible for red blood cells to metabolize normally two chemical components of broad beans, divicine and isouramil, which leads to hemolysis. Glucose-6-phosphate dehydrogenase deficiency, of which there are several variants, is found largely in people of Mediterranean origin, but also African. And, of course, the broad bean is particularly favored in Mediterranean cuisines. It is highly versatile and nutritious, being 25 percent protein by weight, and (very importantly for the authors of the article, who are Italian) delicious. Favism is particularly severe in young children, and is more common in boys, who may suffer a drop in their hemoglobin levels of 50 percent in twenty-four hours, with jaundice and darkened urine. They often have fever and abdominal pain.

The article begins by saying that "Pythagoras of Samos, a great mathematician rather than a physician, may have been the first in stating emphatically, in the 5th century B.C.,[4] that fava beans could be dangerous and even lethal for humans." That seems to me a mistake. The Pythagoreans were forbidden to eat beans, but the reason for this prohibition remains unknown.

---

2 I mean liberal in the old-fashioned European economic sense, not the American self-proclaimed progressive sense.

3 Hemolytic anemia results from the destruction of red blood cells within the body, as against insufficient or deficient production of red cells, or their loss through hemorrhage.

4 Full marks to the authors and editors for not using the mealy-mouthed, cowardly and contemptible B.C.E., Before the Common Era.

The epidemiology of favism makes it very unlikely that Pythagoras would have noticed something that occurs so infrequently, or that he would have made it the reason for a dietary law if he had noticed it. In Sardinia, for example, 958 cases occurred in a population of 500,000 in the years from 1965 through 1979, which amounts to one case per 7,800 of the population per year.[5] The entire population of Greece in the time of Pythagoras would have been similar to that of Sardinia in the fifteen years cited, and as far as is known, he did not travel extensively in Greece. Even if that figure for modern Sardinia is an underestimate (because minor cases do not come to attention), Pythagoras would not have come across very many cases of the sickness. It is improbable that his inevitably tenuous acquaintance with such a condition—even if he recognized its cause—would have been the foundation of so drastic a prohibition. It would be like forbidding people to go into the countryside to avoid snakebites.

Pythagoreanism was an ascetic cult, and it is more likely that the prohibition was related to the bean's deliciousness than to its danger, though possibly its propensity to induce impure flatulence might have played a role. In suggesting that Pythagoras forbade beans, in essence, because of glucose-6-phosphate dehydrogenase deficiency, the authors are following (consciously or not) the doctrines of Marvin Harris, an American social anthropologist of Marxist and Malthusian bent[6] who argued that religious dietary prohibitions had quotidian material reasons behind them, including health reasons. Undercooked pork, for example, can gave rise to cysticercosis and trichinosis, both of them unpleasant and even dangerous, and so there is a "rational" reason underlying the religious prohibition of pork.

This kind of argument rests on what has been called the hermeneutics of suspicion: a belief that the meaning or motive of a human activity is not what the actors say it is but is "really" something that only expert observers armed with a true philosophical anthropology can discern. Thus a man who avoids beans for the sake of his soul is "really" avoiding them because of fear of favism. The purpose of the

---

5 The rate was lower still in a recent report from Gaza.

6 Marx reviled Malthus, but they were at least agreed on the importance of material factors in history.

hermeneutics of suspicion (if I may be allowed to turn its methods on itself) is to portray man as being both utterly earthbound and in principle comprehensible: there is nothing more in heaven and earth than is dreamt of in *your* philosophy.

The authors point out that the dietary information on a prominent self-help website devoted to helping those with glucose-6-phosphate dehydrogenase deficiency is wrong and alarmist. However, alarm is a not altogether disagreeable sensation, certainly not by comparison with boredom.

If our age is the golden age of anything, I should say it is the golden age of the acronym. Of course, it is only other people's acronyms that we object to, our own being used for entirely rational reasons. The problem is that everyone has his perfectly justifiable acronyms, and since we all live in our own little worlds, mutually incomprehensible acronyms proliferate. Sometimes on reading a paper in the *Journal*, I have to keep reminding myself what a previously used acronym stands for. Here is a list, no doubt incomplete, of the acronyms used in this issue:

> ERISA, DAWN, UK, ISSN, TTP, BRCA, DNA, NEJM, JAMA, CBME, ACGME, ABMS, GME, AAMC, UME, EPAC, PBM, HIPAA, IQVIA, H1N1, H3N2, WHO, HA, T160K, CDC, DWI, CTP, CT, NIHSS, MRI, RAPID, SD, CI, NA, UCLA, THRACE, NETT, mRS, EQ-5D, IMS III, DEFUSE 3, USA, ECR, CMAP, mV, msec, BOLD, fMRI, CD34+, DMARD, SCOT, G-CSF, 800 CgY, FVC, DLco, HAQ-DI, SAS, ESR, SF-36, GRCS, mRSS, ASTIS, US, SLS II, ASSIST, NIAID, HALT-MS, CHART-1, EMPOWER, CAFS, CD4+CD25+, HSCT, UTI, CXXR1, H30, ST131, eGFR, IV, ICU, ED, IDSA, SOFA, APACHE, BJU, G6PD, NADPH, NADP, ROS, IgG, HNE, GERD, HIV, VIPoma, PCR, PET, MEN1, PET-CT, MR CLEAN, DWI, CTP, WAKE-UP, ECASS-4 EXTEND, tPA, DIAS-3, DOI, MSLT II, BRAF, MEK, ANZ, DeCOG-SLT, EORTC 18071, HSC, HSCT, BIM, BMF, BCL-XL, TAT-BCL-XL, HLA, MYC, HACA, ADAMTS13, ADA, CR, PR, T2DM, DELIRIUM, FDA, IPTAS, NY, CARS, CME, AMA, PRA.

Some of these are entirely familiar to almost everyone; more are known to every doctor; and each will be familiar to someone. But the overall effect is dizzying. These abbreviations are necessary, but if there is one thing that medicine teaches, to doctors and to patients, it is that the necessary is not necessarily pleasing. ▣

Envoi

I hope to have shown, by this extended commentary on a full year of the *New England Journal of Medicine,* that there is more in a medical journal than straightforward scientific truth, if only because scientific truth is itself often less than straightforward, especially as it approaches the hitherto undiscovered. But I hope also to have shown that, insofar as the *Journal* expresses social attitudes, they are almost all of a certain tendency, which for lack of a better term may be called *politically correct.* Almost no debate on this tendency appears in its pages, as if some power of censorship were at work. (On purely scientific matters, the situation is much better.) Of course, any publication has the right to promote any views it likes and is not under a legal obligation to print anything that it does not like. Still, one might have hoped for lively debate on socially contentious matters in a journal aimed at a highly educated and intelligent audience, who cannot possibly all be of like mind on such issues. The *NEJM* seems to me a manifestation of a dangerous tendency in our society, that of self-enclosure in an ideological laager.

Does this matter very much? How important is the *NEJM?* It is one of the most influential medical journals in the world, but that is not the same as saying that it is very important. After I had finished this book, I spoke to a Dutch surgeon and epidemiologist, working in England, who said to me that in his opinion (which was clearly a very intelligent one) informal sources of information such as personal contact and telephone conversations are actually much more important in the spread of medical advance than journals. And his wife, a distinguished pediatric epidemiologist, warned me that too stringent a criticism of scientific papers, for example by harping on their omissions, risked tearing them out of context; for they were mostly addressed to workers in the field, who would automatically be much more aware of their limitations than a neophyte such as I.

All the same, I cannot help but hope that this book is a contribution to a properly critical attitude to what can so easily, and dangerously, go by default. A critic of the errors of others is a hostage to fortune, since he is bound to make errors of his own,[1] but such are the perils of the intellectual life.

---

1 Which is why the expert witness in trials is well-advised to answer "Yes" or "No," without further elaboration, wherever he can.

Acknowledgments

I should like to thank my friend and colleague, Professor R. E. Ferness for many helpful discussions. He will not agree with all my conclusions, but I hope he will not be offended by them.

I should also like to thank my eagle-eyed editor, Carol Staswick, who saved me from many an error of both style and substance.

All remaining errors are, of course, my own.

Index